Fundamentals of Yoga

Fundamentals of Yoga

A HANDBOOK OF THEORY, PRACTICE, AND APPLICATION

Rammurti S. Mishra, M.D.
(Shri Brahmananda Sarasvati)

Foreword by John White
Introduction by Paul Brunton

Drawings by Oscar Weinland
and Nandini (Lindsay Hutchinson Berté)

HARMONY BOOKS/NEW YORK

Dedicated to my Teacher
Bhagawan Bodhisattwa

Published by Harmony Books, a division of Crown Publishers, Inc., 201 East 50th Street, New York, New York 10022. Member of the Crown Publishing Group.

Random House, Inc. New York, Toronto, London, Sydney, Auckland
www.randomhouse.com

Printed in the United States of America

Library of Congress Cataloging-in-Publication Data
Mishra, Rammurti S.
Fundamentals of yoga / by Rammurti S. Mishra.
1. Yoga. I. Title.
B132.Y6M5 1987 181'.45 86-18460

ISBN 0-517-56422-X

15 14 13 12 11 10 9 8 7

ACKNOWLEDGMENTS

While Yoga is a disciplined, soul-searching path that one must travel alone, I now realize with wonderment and gratitude that it is impossible for me to measure, express, or phrase the thanks I owe my many dear friends in the United States who have made this publication possible. Yoga is many thousands of years old, but the encouragement and enthusiasm of today's American Yoga students inspired this restatement of the age-old truth in today's language against the contemporary scene.

I am especially grateful to The Reverend Dr. Paul Brunton for his gracious introduction of me to Western readers and for reading this book in manuscript. The gentle and wise Dr. Brunton has definitely inherited the mantle of his *guru,* the great Ramana Maharshi.

I am also deeply grateful to my many friends and students of the Yoga Society of New York, Inc., the Yoga Society of Dayton (Ohio), Inc., and the Columbus Yoga Society, Inc., for their faithful co-operation in arranging publishing details, and to Miss Ruth Rohpeter for her generous typing of the manuscript.

I wish to thank The CIBA Pharmaceutical Products, Inc., for their courteous permission to use the wonderful artistry of Dr. Frank H. Netter from the CIBA collection of medical illustrations. The line drawings from these and the other original plates are the talented work of my gifted student, Oscar Weinland.

To Page Newton, my youngest student, I am indebted for his careful execution of the glossary, index, and transliteration.

RAMMURTI S. MISHRA

ACKNOWLEDGMENTS FOR THE 1987 EDITION

I wish to thank all the people over the years who have encouraged and supported efforts to republish *Fundamentals of Yoga,* especially George Leone. Much gratitude goes to Anya Foos-Graber for her tireless follow-through in getting all the pieces of the project together and to Uma Giri, who initiated the renewed efforts. Thanks of course go to the Julian Press for choosing to republish this work for both students of Yoga and the general public. I am grateful to Vyasananda and Radhakrishna (Nicholas Clemente) for the new design and format of this book, as well as to Jan Maupin and all the I.C.S.A. staff.

The new appendix in this edition was created through the combined efforts of Vyasananda and Purnima, who modeled for the Yoga postures; Louis Acker, who photographed them; and Nandini (Lindsay Hutchinson Berté), who reproduced the postures in charming pen and ink drawings. Thanks go to Purnima for her assistance, especially in designing the appendix, again to Jan Maupin for layout, and to Bharati for proofreading the Sanskrit terms.

Thanks also to Ma Chidananda Sarasvati (Mary Tasch, Ph.D.), Sharada (Jill Mellick, Ph.D.), Radha, and Daniel Maziarz for their help. Finally, I wish to thank John White for his thoughtful foreword and Ralph Faillace for the photographic portrait, as well as all the residents of Ananda Ashram.

RAMMURTI S. MISHRA

CONTENTS

ILLUSTRATIONS

FOREWORD

To many Westerners, the word *Yoga* evokes an image of someone twisted like a pretzel or standing on his head chanting strange sounds. Another popularized image of Yoga is a svelte-bodied female who lost thirty pounds and toned up through a Yoga class at the local YMCA. While these images are not inaccurate, they are far from complete as a description of Yoga. They are merely stereotypes, less than half-truths derived from photographs and sensationalized accounts in the media. Newspapers, magazines, books, lecture posters, films, and advertisements have all helped to dramatize and popularize an incomplete picture of what Yoga is.

The truth about Yoga is something far higher and greater. Keenly aware of that, Dr. Rammurti Mishra, in his book, *Fundamentals of Yoga,* offers several striking definitions:

"Yoga is the process of dehypnotism."

"Yoga presents a scientific way and methodical effort to attain perfection through the control of the elements of the physical, metaphysical, and psychical natures."

"Submission of lower desire to higher desire is called Yoga."

"Yoga [is the] great state in which all pains and sufferings are permanently conquered."

"Yoga is mastery of mind."

"Yoga is the foundation of the ethical and moral life upon which the Kingdom of Heaven is established."

The thrust of these statements should indicate to you that Yoga is a lot more than a stylized image of a skinny Indian Yogi, wearing only a loincloth, who has occult powers and bizarre behavior. And it is certainly a lot more than just a system of exercise, relaxation, and weight reduction.

Yoga is probably the most ancient sacred tradition known to humanity. Its roots go back at least 5,000 years, far longer than any other religion or spiritual path. However, Yoga is venerable not simply for its age. It is a time-honored tradition because it has inspected every facet of life, probed it to rock-bottom reality, discovered the secrets there, and offers that knowledge openly to anyone who aspires to attain it. That is, Yoga offers this openly provided that the aspirant recognizes that words alone are not sufficient. There must be practice. There must be direct experience—direct realization of truth.

Yoga has the most sage and yet practical advice for people in all walks of life, of all personalities and professions, in all stages of health or illness, at all levels of education and intelligence. There is nothing—*nothing*—unknown to Yoga. It is all there, waiting for you to grow into it, to discover higher and higher levels of understanding and attainment, until the Secret of Life and the Universe itself—enlightenment—is made plain and obvious.

In short, Yoga is a system for your total development—physically, mentally, and spiritually. The Sanskrit root from which the word comes, *yug,* means "to yoke," "to join," or "to unite." What is united are the individual and the cosmos. Through the methods of Yoga, the individual, to use Dr. Mishra's term, dehypnotizes himself, clears his mind of illusions and unconscious conditioning, so that total mastery of the mind's powers and potentialities is attained. Ultimately, the power and potentiality of our Self is none other than that of the entire cosmos. It is only the ego, the illusion of separate Self, that keeps us from realizing that we are truly divine—truly one with the universe, truly God in human form.

The practice of Yoga, then, is both the means and the goal. Yoga has developed many branches or lines that differ from one another in emphasis or methodology. But theoretically, all of them lead to the same condition, which is known as *moksha,* meaning "liberation," or "enlightenment." And what is liberation, or enlightenment? To quote Dr. Mishra again, "*Moksha,* or *nirvanam,* is the permanent abode of eternal consciousness. Knowledge, existence, blessings, happiness, and peace—Yoga is the infallible instrument to attain *nirvanam.* Thus, the main goal of Yoga is freedom of the spirit from the fetters of material desires and permanent victory of consciousness over ignorance."

Fundamentals of Yoga can be a valuable resource for those seeking to find their true Self in the context of daily living. I am, therefore, happy to recommend the book as a guide to the true perspective and practices of Yoga.

JOHN WHITE,
Editor of *Frontiers of Consciousness*
and *What Is Enlightenment?*

INTRODUCTION

Dr. Mishra is a successful physician and surgeon, professor of medicine in R. A. Podar Medical College, Bombay, India, and chief physician to M. A. Podar Hospital, attached to the same medical college. To interpret yogic anatomy and physiology, yogic psychology, and the psychic centers (*cakras*) in modern terminology, he has performed 1,348 autopsies.

In addition he has done research work in endocrinology, modern psychology, and other branches of medicine in European and American medical institutions as well as in those of India, his own country. All this has been linked to the expert knowledge of *rāja* Yoga, of which he is both a theoretical student and a working practitioner. He has used it to illuminate references in the Yoga texts dealing with such anatomic and physiologic obscurities as *kuṇḍalinī, suśumna, pingalà,* etc. He has brilliantly joined together the deep relaxation techniques of Yoga with the therapeutic and psychological techniques of the art of suggestion, which was made familiar to us by Coué and the New Thought cults. He has effected a similar conjunction between Yoga and Vedānta. He has explained simply and directly the breathing, gazing, and other exercises used as aids to mind control.

Two famous teachers exerted a profound influence on Dr. Mishra's spiritual perceptions: Shankaracharya Shri Shankara, Purushottama Teerthaji, Leader of Sahja Yoga Movement, Sidha Yogashram, Banaras; and Baba Soma Natha, Leader of Radha-Swami Movement, Bombay.

Subsequently, still in search of his ultimate *guru,* he traveled around the circle of Indian *āśrams,* but, until he met a mysterious person who disdained publicity, deliberately confined his instruction to a few selected students, and was known only to a small circle, did not feel himself in the presence of a Yogi whose development was full enough. In this great man, whose name was Bhagavandas, Dr. Mishra found the full vision of *nirvāṇam* and an inexpressible magnetic influence radiating from him. He chose him as his teacher. The *guru's* original home is still unknown. In his younger days he was in Karachi, but during the violent upheaval that separated Pakistan from India he came to visit his beloved disciples in India and at their earnest request was persuaded to remain there. When he left his body in 1957, in Bombay, he was over 100 years old but looked much younger.

In admirable contrast to much of the excessively theoretical, mainly metaphysical, or merely platitudinous writing in this field, these pages abound in working methods and exercises for use by the earnest student who seeks to spiritualize himself. Altogether, they constitute a fascinating volume for all those interested in the subject.

PAUL BRUNTON

PREFACE

Through innumerable incarnations and rebirths man has hypnotized himself with his body. Because of his own ignorance he feels that his Self and consciousness are limited to his body. When, through the practice of Yoga, his ignorance is destroyed and he removes his hypnotism of finiteness, the Self, which is infinite and does not admit of any multiplicity whatsoever, reveals itself by itself, like the sun when the clouds are removed. The notion of man, woman, animal, god, child, youth, and age is superimposed upon the Self by ignorance. Yoga is the process of dehypnotism. By means of contemplation, concentration, and meditation, one realizes the true form of the Self, which is omnipresence, omnipotence, and omniscience.

In my long journey, thousands have asked me these questions: "How do you practice *samādhi*? How do you go into the state of enlightenment and *nirvāṇam*? Could I learn to practice *samādhi*? Could I attain the state of enlightenment and *nirvāṇam*?" To the first and second questions I answer: "*Samādhi* is based on fixation, suggestion, and will power on the part of the operator, and the state of enlightenment and *nirvāṇam* depends on *prajñā, śīla,* and *samādhi* (intuition, ethical and moral perfection, and constant concentration)." To the fourth question I reply: "Yes, you too can become an expert student of Yoga and can attain the state of enlightenment and *nirvāṇam* by learning the laws of the mind and nature, and the simple laws of *samādhi*." Perfection is not an accidental phenomenon and it is not a monopoly of any particular nation or a particular person. He who practices concentration, obtains it.

Since the prehistoric era, man has known and used Yoga *samādhi* and obtained enlightenment and *nirvāṇam*. During this time, much has been written on the Yoga science, the material on the eternal science of Yoga perhaps forming the greatest library on any single subject. There are many people throughout the world who are interested in learning the science of Yoga. Also, there are many books on Yoga being sold in the market today. Many of these books are supposed to be instructive as textbooks to teach you "How to go into the state of *samādhi* and how to attain enlightenment and perfection." Most of these books only pretend to do so but do not "teach you how," because they present a great number of useless theories, dogmas, and various other window dressings to "load" their pages, but you are not interested in useless verbiage to waste your valuable time. You want to know "how." This book will explain to you "how."

To the man educated in modern universities in the East or West, the scheme of Yoga and Vedānta to attain perfection appears to be only an elaborate process of self-hypnotism. No doubt some modern fanatical mendicants and professional Yogis and practitioners of the *tantra* cult are the main cause of confusion, but the Patañjalī Yoga in its original form is free from these vagaries. Therefore, the name of the Patañjalī Yoga is *Sāṃkhya* Yoga. The main reason for this name is that the Patañjalī Yoga does not recognize physics without metaphysics and, vice versa, metaphysics without physics. It is the missing link between the two sciences, hence the name is *Sāṃkhya* Yoga (Vedānta with practice, knowledge through experience). It is the king of all Yogas; therefore it is called *Rāja* Yoga. As mathematics is the root of all physical sciences, so the *sāṃkhya* system is the root of metaphysical science.

Each and every soul is potentially divine but, owing to ignorance, it is not in its real form. Yoga adopts all those possible forms of practice which actualize its divinity, and gives full freedom to all students to adopt other methods to develop will power and the thinking process according to time and personal situations. Thus, it is free from the dogmatism, orthodoxism, and conservatism of all religions of the world. Yoga is not a branch of any particular religion but helps every religion in the right way.

By practicing the methods and formulas of Yoga, one brings one's innermost consciousness up from the deeper levels to the functional levels. This inner consciousness is the reservoir of all life. Each body is a divine instrument.

It is the eternal transmitter and receiver. Sense organs are conceived as receivers and motor organs as transmitters. The mind is controller of both. Although every living being, from the one-cellular to the multicellular, has the power of transmission and of reception, nevertheless it is evoluted in higher stages and involuted in lower stages. Hence, the "normal" limits of human vision are his own limitation; they are neither universal nor natural nor ultimate, but they are individual, unreal, and temporary. Through the discipline of body, senses, and mind, *cittam* is purified for the beatific vision of the soul, and the student realizes that the real intelligence and memory are independent of the cerebral mechanism. The human mind has perceptive faculties other than those served by the five senses. The five senses which we share with the lower animals are common to all, but through practice of *samādhi,* other worlds are revealed that are uncommon and eternal. Once the real eyes of the student are opened, he has an extension of his perception as stupendous as that of a previously blind man when he first acquires sight.

There are laws of supreme nature and supreme consciousness governing the acquisition of this larger vision and the manifestation of latent powers. By following the principles of Yoga, one heightens the power of concentration, arrests the vagaries of the mind by fixing one's attention on different *cakras,* and one masters one's soul in the same way as an athlete masters his body. One can acquire the power of seeing and knowing without the help of other senses and can become independent of the activities one exercises through the physical senses and the brain.

Thus, Yoga presents a scientific way and methodical effort to attain perfection through the control of the elements of the physical, metaphysical, and psychical natures. The physical body, the active will power, and the understanding mind are brought under perfect control, which leads to spiritual freedom. The aim of Yoga is not to formulate metaphysical theories, but to formulate the practical method of indicating "how" salvation can be attained by disciplined mind.

Since the life of man depends on the nature of the mind-stuff (*cittam*), purification of the mind-stuff is extremely necessary through concentration of mental waves. Since the practice of Yoga depends on *sāṃkhya* philosophy, the table of *sāṃkhya* metaphysics will be useful to remember before going into concentration.

This table will help the student to reach a higher level of consciousness through a transformation of the gross and multiple universe and the body into *pañca mahābūta* (five states of atomic nature and consciousness); *pañca mahābhūta* into *pañca tanmātra* (five prenuclear states of nature and consciousness); organs of perception, organs of action, and *pañca tanmātra* (five prenuclear states) into universal ego (*ahaṃkāra*); the universal ego into universal *mahat tatva* (universal intelligence); universal intelligence into supreme nature and supreme consciousness.

The Self is one-without-a-second. Supreme nature is no longer a separate principle in liberation, but it is the eternal energy of prime *puruṣa* by which the *puruṣa* projects, protects, and involutes the multiple universe.

The cause of suffering is ignorance. Dualism is due to ignorance. This dualism is removed when ignorance is removed by *samādhi*. The multiple world with its dualism disappears for a liberated man and he obtains *nirvāṇam*, the true form of the spirit.

Now you are about to begin your course. I will give you all the principles and theories that you shall need, but I have eliminated all those principles and theories which are beyond the approach of beginners. Principles and theories described herein are the "essence" of all theories and principles. By practicing these, you will understand later on all theories and principles, and you will formulate your own theories and principles.

There is nothing I have written in the pages of this book that cannot be proved according to the objective criteria of modern science. Medical doctors, biologists, psychologists, and physicists have encountered many of these data in their own research and have validated their actuality and potential. At present their interest flows along other lines and they are not yet ready to utilize more fully these natural phenomena; it is unquestionable, however, that although modern science and Yoga seem to travel different roads, their goals are similar.

What should also be kept in view is that I am a medical doctor and a scientist of the twentieth century and that my standards must be rather demanding; if I prefer the methods and philosophy of Yoga to other existing means, it is because I have found them to be the most practical way of expressing myself and my knowledge.

I promise to make this course very brief but I also promise to give you every known successful and practical method of *rāja* Yoga that has been tested and proved by innumerable brilliant scholars of Yoga over many thousands of years of practice; to help make you a successful student of Yoga and to recognize your master, your innermost soul, your eternity, your freedom, your liberation, your *nirvāṇam,* presently unknown to you, but a companion and comrade to you.

In the following chapters I will give you the basic and primary principles of Yoga psychology and Yoga *samādhi,* giving you the keys to unlock the doors that stand between you and your master, the eternal mind.

Thirty lessons are devoted to this purpose. Do not read this like a novel but read one lesson, understand it, enlarge it by your commentary, consult anatomic, physiologic, and Yoga psychologic pictures and references prescribed with the lessons, concentrate according to it, and then start the next lesson. If you practice meditation, concentration, and contemplation this way, success will be the by-product of your practice and it will remain with you permanently.

With these terms I wish good luck and a good future to every living being.

PREFACE TO THE 1987 EDITION

The latest discoveries of medical science and psychology are pointing us in the direction of the ancient science of Yoga. Medical science increasingly shows us that most physical diseases are psychosomatic in origin; they begin in the mind—that is to say, with man's disconnection from Nature. Psychology, especially humanistic annd transpersonal psychology, is uncovering the mind's incredible abilities to heal and develop "paranormal" powers. We are on the verge of another gigantic leap in human evolution. We will learn to tap and utilize our great inner powers to create peace on Earth.

For thousands of years, the Yogis of India have used the classical methodologies of their science to heal their bodies and expand their consciousness. For many decades now, Westerners have also practiced these methods with success. Meditation is now prescribed for patients suffering from high blood pressure and other ailments. In the "First Surgeon General's Report on Health Promotion and Disease Prevention," public health authorities declared that to improve our health significantly, we must improve our lifestyle and explore the use of nontraditional medical means. The government also now recommends a more Yogic diet for Americans, one including less fat and meat and more fresh fruits, vegetables, and grains. Because Americans are responding to this call, the rate of heart disease and cancer is dropping.

All these developments are quite heartening to me. When I first wrote *Fundamentals of Yoga* in 1959, I was a pioneer in the field. The techniques and practice of Yoga had not been explored from the scientific and medical point of view. Now this approach has become popular with many professionals. Thousands of people have benefited from using *Fundamentals of Yoga*.

My goal is to demystify Yoga, to show that it is a practical science that can dramatically improve the physical, mental, and spiritual well-being of any person who chooses to use it. Yoga is not a religion, therefore it can be practiced in partnership with any religious belief. What is the religion of earth, water, fire, air, the sun, the moon, the stars, and space? They have no particular religion; these belong to all humanity.

Yoga is beyond religion. Yoga belongs to everybody. It may be thought of as the cosmic religion. All religions use symbols in the form of language. Yoga deals directly with Ultimate Reality, pure awareness, pure consciousness, beyond the body and mind, beyond time and space. The founders of all religions simply observed and experienced this same cosmic religion in their own way, in their own times.

One who uses the mind, the psyche, properly in time and space with an unselfish motive for the common welfare of humankind is a Yogi and is practicing Yoga. Yoga is the holistic way of life, in which the union and harmony of the body, mind, and soul, or consciousness (the "I-am"), are fundamental. Therefore, Yoga has many branches that are contained in four main groups: physical Yoga, mental Yoga, spiritual Yoga, and special Yoga.

1. *Physical Yoga:* Hatha Yoga embodies a variety of physical exercises, or *asanas.* There are cosmetic, therapeutic, relaxing, and meditative effects to Hatha Yoga. Other forms of physical Yoga include dance, running, jogging, and swimming Yoga; walking-together Yoga; natural food and cooking Yoga; work or karma Yoga; occupational Yoga; Yoga for all senior citizens to make their lives happy; in short, Yoga as a natural way of life, including natural birth, life, sickness, and natural death. Each of these forms of Yoga is practiced according to one's ability. Yet this is not a complete list. It is only meant to indicate that each of life's activities when performed in a natural, harmonious way unites the body, mind, and spirit; that is to say, to create perfect balance is a Yoga.
2. *Mental Yoga:* Whatever you can do with your mind is called mental Yoga. Mental Yoga works psychologically and pathologically. Psychologically, it reveals all layers of the mind: the conscious, subconscious, unconscious, collective unconscious, and superconscious levels. It also removes anxiety, jealousy, depression, confusion, ignorance, and hate, and brings perfection to the mind through concentration. Mental Yoga includes mantra Yoga (*man* means "mind," and *tra* means "protection"; anything that protects the mind and helps it to go up and up is called mantra); meditation Yoga; sankirtan and bha-

jan Yoga; painting, sculpture, tea and flower ceremony Yoga; music, theater, dance, and writing Yoga, etc. The treatment of the individual psyche, or individual "I-am," by means of the cosmic psyche, or the universal "I-am", is mental Yoga and is leading to the development of new forms of psychotherapy, psychoanalysis, depth psychology, transpersonal psychology, psychosynthesis, and consciousness research.

3. *Spiritual Yoga:* The union of the individual "I-am" with the cosmic, universal "I-am" is spiritual Yoga. Laya Yoga, Integral Yoga, and Raja Yoga can also be considered spiritual Yoga.
4. *Special Yoga:* This final group includes tantra Yoga, yantra Yoga, and kriya Yoga. Tantra Yoga is the union of conscious and unconscious energy (*Purusha* and *Prakriti*). Yantra Yoga is the mechanism of expression of conscious and unconscious energy through the symbolism of mandala, geometry, architecture, etc. Kriya Yoga is the Yoga of transformation of the individual "I-am" into the universal "I-am."

Yoga is balance of the mind—individually, domestically, socially, nationally, internationally, and cosmologically—with benefits for all.

What is the difference between science and Yoga? Science deals with objective reality, while Yoga begins with subjective reality and ends in transcendental reality. Science is busy with all types of discoveries and inventions, while Yoga is mainly interested in the discovery of the discoverer—the discovery of pure awareness, pure consciousness, Absolute "I-am." When you have Self, pure consciousness, and pure awareness, then you know the whole universe, whether objective or subjective, past, present, or future. Then, truly, you are beyond time and space.

History tells us that within the last 3,000 years we have had more than 5,000 religious wars! Earth is suffering from crisis, disorder, confusion, disharmony, pollution, nuclear threat, hijacking, terrorism, and mistrust between East and West. We have the choice between death and life. If we prefer to die, then we do not have to do anything. But if we prefer to live, then we have to change our hearts completely. This transformation cannot be done without Yoga or similar practices that lead one to experience inner and outer unity.

Our hearts are for unity, and our brains are for multiplicity. We need both, integrated harmoniously. This is not the job of the United Nations or any national government. Nature is already working toward natural union and natural multiplicity. If we do not disturb the work of nature, then nature will lead us toward our perfection. Separated from nature's cosmic religion, we die; united, we live.

The practice of Yoga as a way of life can assist us in achieving inner and outer unity. Yoga is our universal common-wealth.

KEY TO TRANSLITERATION OF YOGIC SANSKRIT TERMS

In the case that the student of Yoga is interested in learning the correct pronunciation of Yogic terminology, or a near approximation of it, all terms in the text have been rendered into the standard system of transliteration, a key tc which is given below:

VOWELS

A- as in but
Ā- as in father
I- as in become
Ī- as in seat
U- as in put
Ū- as in cool
E- as in French beau
AI- as in nice
O- as in Fench beau
AU- as in house
ṚI- similar to Spanish 'rr' (cerebral)
Ḷ similar to Ṛ, but dental

CONSONANTS

Ṃ- resonant nasal sound after a vowel
Ḥ- emphasized 'hard' breath after a vowel
K,P- as in English, but with less aspiration
C- similar to the English 'ch'
Ṭ- similar to the English 't', with tongue bent back to touch the roof of palate
T- tongue touching upper teeth
KH, CH, ṬH, TH, PH,- close union of respective consonant with aspiration 'h', e.g. KH as in Lakehouse
G- as in go
J- as in English
B- as in English
Ḍ,D- soft (voiced) equivalents of Ṭ,T
GH, JH, ḌH, DH, BH- soft equivalents of the above aspirates
Ṅ- as in think
Ñ- as in angel
Ṇ- peculiar nasal sound,with tongue rolled back to touch roof of palate
N- tongue touching teeth
M- as in English
Y- as in yes
R- as in Spanish pero
L- tongue touching teeth
V- usually like English v, after consonants, more like English w
Ś- like English sh
Ṣ- similar to Ś but with tongue in 'cerebral' position
S,H- as in English
JÑ- like nasalized 'gy', or also, 'jy'

TREE OF SĀṂKHYA

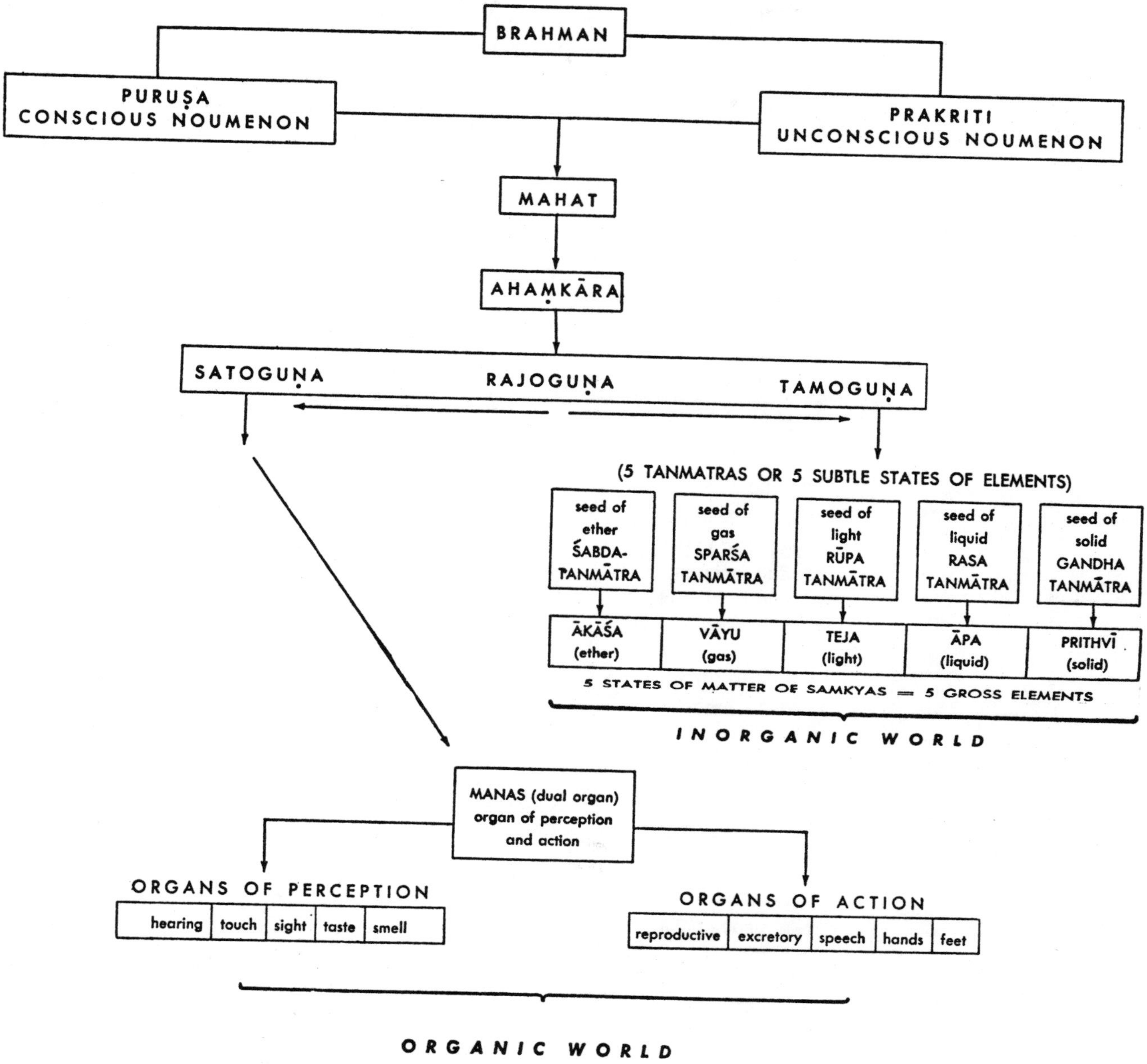

Brahman— Ultimate Reality, Truth
Prakṛiti— Primordial energy, Unconscious Unconditional
Puruṣa— Cosmic consciousness (unconditional)
Mahat— Cosmic intelligence (conditional)
Ahaṃkāra— Universal ego, Self-consciousness
Manas— Mind

COSMIC FORCES OF NATURE:
Satoguṇa— Light, Intelligence
Rajoguṇa— Active state of the mind
Tamoguṇa—Force of Equilibrium

Cittam— Mind (Manus) plus Ego (Ahaṃkāra) plus Intelligence (Mahat)
Citi— Puruṣa

1

YOGA AND ITS APPLICATION

Submission of lower desire to higher desire is called Yoga. In Yoga the student leads his mind from untruth to truth, from darkness to light, from ignorance to knowledge, from pain, sufferings, diseases, and death to peace, happiness, and eternity, from unreality to reality.

Yoga teaches the methods to control the mighty waves of the mind and to subdue them completely to the primordial consciousness, which is operating eternally through every perceptual mechanism. It is working as eternal teacher for the student of Yoga. Without understanding this principle, Yoga practice is impossible.

Yoga does not recognize physics without metaphysics or metaphysics without physics. Thus, Yoga is a missing link between physics and metaphysics; it criticizes both when they try to become separate and brings them together into one eternal principle, which is called *ultimate reality*.

Many people learn Yoga, some to conquer their physical and mental illness, and weakness, while others learn it to obtain some occult powers. Philosophers learn Yoga to make alive their philosophy, because without the practice of Yoga, the teachings of philosophy and Vedānta are like a lifeless body. Religious persons practice methods of Yoga to perceive truth in the scriptural statements, because without the practice of Yoga, all scriptures are nothing but figurative statements. Hypnotists learn Yoga in the form of hypnotism (a distorted form of Yoga), to become professional hypnotists. Some learn Yoga as a curiosity, while a few learn Yoga for the sake of tremendous magical powers.

While Yoga definitely has all the above-mentioned powers, its real aim is beyond these goals. Once the first writer of Yoga Sutras—Patañjalī—was asked by his student: "Sir, you have written a book of medicine which treats mental and physical diseases temporarily. Is there any way to conquer mental and physical illnesses, pains, sufferings, and death permanently?" The great Yogi Patañjalī replied as follows:

"Yoge mokṣe ca sarveṣām vedanānām avartam mokṣe nirvṛittiḥ niḥśeṣa Yogomokṣa pravartakaḥ"—that is to say, Yoga and Mokṣaḥ are two great states in which all pains and sufferings are permanently conquered. Mokṣaḥ or *nirvāṇam* is the permanent abode of eternal consciousness. Knowledge, existence, blessings, happiness, and peace—Yoga is the infallible instrument to obtain *nirvāṇam*. Thus, the main goal of Yoga is freedom of the spirit from the fetters of material desires and permanent victory of consciousness over ignorance. With the exception of *nirvāṇam*, all other perfections, such as mysticism, occult powers, supernatural powers, etc., are secondary aims and they are by-products of Yoga. A student of Yoga is constantly warned about the use of these powers, because in his demonstration of powers he may fall from his highest aim, which is complete victory of consciousness over ignorance and nature. He is allowed to use his "supernatural" powers of Yoga if their use is not contrary to his ultimate goal. This is the main difference between a student of Yoga and other mystics. If someone is not interested in perfection, but only to gain some "supernatural" powers, he can still practice Yoga, but he must understand clearly that this is not the true form of Yoga.

Some religionists try to associate the science of Yoga with religions; it is a misapplication of Yoga. No doubt the methods of Yoga help all religions equally in their practice of meditation, yet Yoga is beyond religion. It comprises every science, still it is beyond all sciences. It has its own methods of investigating mental powers; other scientific investigations are secondary to Yoga. All other scientific investigations help in the analysis of thought, but one should not forget to analyze the mind through the methods of Yoga practice, which is the direct way of analysis. Yoga is not the property of any country, as some writers claim; it is the property of nature and consciousness, which belongs to everybody equally.

Yoga is used to cure all physical and mental illness with absolute safety and without any harm. Yoga is a simple, easy-to-learn science. Like all sciences, it is founded on facts investigated through analysis and synthesis of thoughts. Yoga consists of analysis of both subject and object, while all other sciences analyze object only. In the state of meditation, the mind is tremendously brighter, stronger, and is possessed of far greater command of all organs and senses. Yoga is mastery of mind. To achieve this purpose, one has to be alert to every branch of science, because directly or indirectly they are all by-products of thoughts.

This course serves as the official text of the school where the average student (class or private) begins practice of the subject at the very first lesson.

The methods contained herein have been tested and proved. With this course you have everything in your possession to become a Yogi, a master of mind. Study these methods, use them, test them, prove them.

CAUTION: In a very short time, as a result of the practice prescribed in this course, you may be able to cure your diseases and weaknesses, mental or physical. Do not attempt to cure anybody of anything. Leave curing to medical practitioners. They are well aware of the powers of Yoga.

Now you are going to learn the principles of Yoga and their application to your mind, senses, and body. From a practical point of view, Yoga is classified into the following eight systems:

1. *Yama* — Control of the mind and mental waves.
2. *Niyama* — Observation of rules to obtain that aim.
3. *Āsana* — Different postures to obtain that state.
4. *Prāṇāyāma* — Regular breathing to help control of mind.
5. *Pratyāhāra* — Complete relaxation of every organ and withdrawal of consciousness.
6. *Dhāraṇā* — Fixation of consciousness on different parts of the body.
7. *Dhyāna* — Constant suggestions.
8. *Samādhi* — Creation of will power, and power of consciousness.

Out of these eight, the last three are primary to mental analysis, and five are secondary to these three. A detailed description of all these will be given later on in your practice. At this time you must learn a few points seriously:

1. Confidence: You must have tremendous confidence in yourself that you can do anything suggested and given to you.
2. Expectation: Whatever is suggested is going to happen.
3. Continuous suggestions.
4. Remove wanderings of the mind at the time of practice so that you may perform your practice fully.
5. Constant remembrance of eternal consciousness, which is operating in you through your heart, and which is manifested in you as your eternal companion and teacher to teach you, and to deliver you from all bondages. It is manifested in you in the form of different divine sounds—*anāhat nādam*—a subtle and constant inexpressible musical vibration in your head, an almost humming sound similar to the pronounced word OM. If it is not manifested in you, do not worry, as it will come in time. If you have it already, use it now in suggested methods.

2
THE POWER OF SUGGESTION: DHĀRAṆĀ, DHYĀNA, AND SAMĀDHI

The universe is governed by eternal laws that never fail. These eternal laws are governed by the suggestion of primordial consciousness. This suggestion is operating in every being, living or nonliving, at all times, in all places, in all experiences, and in all stages of nature, whether it is phenomenon or noumenon, manifested or unmanifested. Therefore, it is extremely necessary that the student of Yoga have an understanding of these laws.

Eight steps or systems of Yoga are mentioned in the first lesson. The last three of them, *dhāraṇā* (fixation of the mind in a particular place, outside or inside the body), *dhyāna* (suggestion), and *samādhi* (development of will power and intuition) are vitally needed for the attainment of supreme consciousness. Therefore, these three are called the internal instrument of consciousness, and the first five are called the external instrument. When one has obtained the form of supreme consciousness, these three, too, become secondary to consciousness.

Suggestion is the most important of these three. Suggestion is the underlying and fundamental cause of all mental phenomena and is the powerful instrument of *samādhi*. The whole universe is nothing but suggestion; the world lives by it. The greatest power of nature is the power of suggestion. It is as old as nature and as powerful as nature. We are constantly moving every moment by our suggestion. First we think, then we do. First we plan, then we accomplish that plan. The newborn baby is not able to walk like a young child; it gives constant suggestion to its body through the mind and after one or two years' practice of suggestion and of trial it becomes able to walk like a man.

Knowledge or anything that we know now has come to us through the power of suggestion. In school, in college, and in universities we learn through the suggestion of our teachers. All newborn babies are ignorant. During their childhood, teens, and adult life they develop themselves according to suggestions that they receive through external and internal surroundings. Through constant suggestion, the same child becomes master of his subject. Any knowledge that we are acquiring at present or that which we expect to acquire in the future will come to us through the power of suggestion.

Even the knowledge that seems to be spontaneous to you is manifested to you by the power of suggestion from the primordial creative energy, Universal Mind, the omniscience, omnipotence, omnipresence, the Universal Intelligence of the supreme. All knowledge was here before you and this universe were born, and it will remain here forever, after you and the universe are gone. And so will the great power of suggestion.

The law of suggestion is infallible and absolute. Everybody, ignorant or wise, rich or poor, high or low, young or old, organic or inorganic, living or nonliving being is subservient to the power and law of suggestion. There is no exception to this law. It is not a respecter of man or monkey, with the sole exception of those who have fortified themselves with the law of suggestion, with divine will power. All suggestions take effect sooner or later. We develop our good or bad life according to our constant suggestion. Suggestion is the greatest single factor in the practice of Yoga. Without understanding the science and methods of suggestion, nobody could obtain perfection of consciousness.

The following are the forms of suggestions:

1. Physical Suggestion: Our body is moved with every thought in a particular way. When someone addresses a meeting, his hands are moving accordingly. By the suggestions of his hands and face, he may express his thoughts in a better way than those who do not show any gesture or physical suggestion to their audience. These and other similar expressions are called physi-

cal suggestion. However, in Yoga physical suggestions are deeper than this. They are different—*mudras* (movements of limbs and fingers, etc., according to the circulation of *kuṇḍalinī* force, magnetic force in the body). Physical suggestions are innumerable and every suggestion is related to a particular type of mental development. You will know them in time by your own experience in the practice of Yoga.

2. Suggestions of Senses: We constantly give and receive suggestions through our sense organs. Children recognize anger or love for them through their parents' eyes. We read written suggestions through the eyes and hear lectures in school and college through the ear. We smell pleasant or unpleasant odor through the nose, know touch and temperature through the skin. These and other similar suggestions are called suggestions of the senses.
3. Verbal Suggestion: This is a special type of suggestion. Through this medium we repeat our ideas and thoughts and achieve success in time. Teachers teach their students through verbal suggestion. You become aware of numberless varieties of verbal suggestions.
4. Mental Suggestion: When a suggestion is repeated only by the mind it is called mental suggestion. The mental suggestion is the strongest of all.
5. Environmental Suggestion: According to the state of the external and internal world, we receive and respond to environmental suggestion. No one can stand extreme heat or cold without proper protection to the body; this is an example of environmental suggestion.
6. Autosuggestion: That suggestion which students of Yoga give to themselves to attain perfection in this practice.

Through the different types of suggestion we direct mental power and thoughts that are the foundation of all suggestions. No one speaks a word, makes a gesture, without its being the result of thought. Speaking and acting are merely accessory to thoughts and indicate what you are thinking. Therefore, all suggestions are the prolongation of mental suggestions. They spring from the mind and dissolve into the mind again. Mental suggestion is the foundation of all suggestions and it is independent. Therefore, in perfection, mental suggestion works without the rest. All other suggestions are dependent and cannot operate without the mind. When you have controlled your mind and mental waves up to a certain extent, and when the magnetic force of your mind radiates through your face, which is the index of your inner success, the people with whom you are in contact come under the influence of this magnetic force, forget their pain, suffering, and anxiety, and become peaceful and calm. They conquer their weakness and, according to their preparation, develop will power in themselves. When people watch you perform Yoga activity and other daily work happily, they too will tend to become perfectly calm without your speaking to them. This is because, when you gaze at certain types of people who are sincere and enthusiastic, waves of your mind pass to them to awaken their minds. They feel this influence and recognize that you enlighten their minds. They feel that you are helping them, protecting them, and guiding them, and eventually they become Yogis and obtain perfection in their practice. That is why people run from *guru* to *guru* and teacher to teacher to obtain "mental" strength from the teacher. This is mental suggestion.

Mental suggestions are as real as the universe around you. Thoughts are things and things are thoughts. Energy is created by the mind and controlled by the mind, and vice versa. The greatest force in the world is mental suggestion. Mind is universe and universe is manifestation of Universal Mind. Mind is matter and all material things are only an expression of the mind.

Mental waves, thought waves, mental force, thought force do not recognize cause, effect, space, and time. They are beyond the causal group. Your mind waves can influence the stars a million miles away. In a moment you can send your thought to a person who is far away from you. You can know past events and future incidents in the same way that you see different countries on maps open before you. You can receive these supernatural powers by the practice of Yoga. Your mind, through the practice of Yoga, can be transformed into an eternal transmitter and receiver. It can work in you like an eternal broadcasting station. When you read a book, magazine, or newspaper, when you see anything, touch anything, smell anything, hear anything, do anything, it is mental suggestion that is performing everything. Still, it is unknown to you. When mental suggestion is not with you, you cannot listen to a radio or to a lecture, to a concert, or to an individual speaking. You can do nothing when it is not with you. When you see a thing, reason about it, and recognize it, mental suggestion is operating in every process. So you see you can be reading, discussing philosophical or other matters in your mind, searching different answers, applying different logics, comparing different states of possibilities, doing everything with your mind, and yet the mind does not speak to you in that way in which we speak to one another. Mental suggestion in these states is without verbal suggestion. Mental suggestion takes the form of other suggestion in later states.

Environmental suggestion is very important in mental development. To environ means to surround, to be around, to hem in; mental means the mind. Any suggestion that is around the mind and creating its impression within the mind is called environmental suggestion. It plays a most important part in the success of meditation and concentration. Natural scenes—waterfalls, oceans, rivers, and forests—have most significant influence over the mind. This is the reason why great Yogis select natural scenes for their meditation. Beginners should go, now and then, to any mountainous place full of natural beauty for a few days' or months' practice of meditation. Even the most restless mind is influenced by it. Beginners should examine their environment if they are not successful in their meditation and select a better one.

The suggestion that a student repeats to his own consciousness is called autosuggestion. It may be verbal, mental, or environmental. There is one other variety of autosuggestion. It is called spontaneous suggestion. It is not necessarily in the operator. It might be verbal, mental, or environmental, but mainly it emerges from the operator; hence it is part of autosuggestion. Some regard it as a separate class. Auto means self. Suggestion means presenting an idea to the mind directly: by word, tone, look, or by external and internal surroundings. Autosuggestion, therefore, means talking to yourself and suggesting to yourself. Autosuggestion is the principal part of concentration.

When teachers teach Yoga, it is suggestion, and when they meditate themselves, it is autosuggestion. Autosuggestion is the life of meditation.

There is one eternal fact: Either you always receive suggestions from your mind or you command your mind by your own suggestion. The moment you are careless, your mind governs you by suggestion. This is called bondage and weakness. But if you command your mind constantly, it will obey you. This is freedom. *Samādhi* depends on autosuggestion. In bondage, people are subservient to the suggestions of their minds and consequently they suffer. All suggestions must be subservient to autosuggestion. They should be allowed if they are not in contradiction to autosuggestion, and they must be checked immediately if they contradict it. Autosuggestion is always immediate, dynamic incentive to *samādhi* or other action.

When a mental wave is projected from the subconscious mind it is called suggestion, and when this mental wave is accepted in the form of an idea, image, or an impulse of thought, it becomes a part of conscious mind and part of individual personality. Now an individual acts and reacts accordingly. Now it is patent mental force that is growing to produce a good or bad habit, according to the variety of autosuggestion. All suggestions, whether mental, verbal, or environmental, operate through autosuggestion. Therefore, all suggestion is autosuggestion. A man cannot perform any work about which he has not made suggestion to himself. When people are suffering from pain, disease, and anxiety, it means they have invited these to become part of their autosuggestion. Yogis advise the student of Yoga not to give any destructive suggestion to his mind. Most people suffer from destructive suggestions which they have already given in the form of thought and image to their minds, and Yogis are happy and calm because they always give divine suggestions to their minds.

Suggestion Is the Key to Meditation. No suggestion, no meditation; evil suggestion, unhappy life; good suggestion, happy life.

First, suggestion is presented to the mind in the form of idea, thought, reason, philosophy. Then it descends to the plane of senses and speech. From the stage of senses and speech it descends into the organs of action and takes the form of action. And now man is according to his action.

Thus, suggestion has four stages:

1. State of mind: To think, to reason, and the like.
2. State of speech: To form ideas.
3. State of action: To form action.
4. State of being and becoming.

Before it bursts into full-fledged action, it remains in the subconscious mind, like electromagnetic force, and when it descends to the conscious mind, it becomes "thought force," "philosophy," "principle," "knowledge," etc. Still, it is limited by individual qualifications. When it ascends into the superconscious state of mind through *samādhi,* it becomes universal force, supreme consciousness, eternal magnetic force.

Autosuggestion is the greatest energy of all, and it is the greatest of all cures. By it a man can alleviate, minimize, eliminate fear of pain, fear of torture, fear of suffering, mental conflicts, and ultimately he can conquer death and may obtain freedom and liberation from all bondages. Even beginners in Yoga can remove any physical and mental disorder by autosuggestion.

Many people suffer because by their destructive autosuggestions they have hypnotized themselves into their conditions. By the process of Yoga, people have to remove that hypnotic state from their minds and must establish a natural state of mind, a normal, healthy condition. Yoga is dehypnotism. People are the architects of their own sufferings, as well as victims of unfortunate autosuggestions. These unfortunate and disastrous autosuggestions are going on in the minds of everyone, and many modern movies, television, stories, and the like aid negative autosuggestions. Fortunate persons control these evil suggestions and fill their minds with divine and meritorious autosuggestions.

By autosuggestion a beginner should re-establish confidence in his mind. Thus, he will be able to conquer his sufferings, fears, phobias, and other conscious and unconscious mental waves. It is the aim of this course to train the beginner to control his mental and physical pains, sufferings, and diseases and to enjoy living with eternal consciousness. This course presents a special technique of concentration in sufficient detail and clarity so that both the beginner and the advanced student may enrich himself at the early stages with divine and eternal virtues.

Sit down comfortably on the ground or in an easy chair. First remember your mind and mental power. Salute all divine seers, teachers, and Yogis; be ready to accept what is truth and beneficial, and to renounce what is untruth and injurious. Begin *dhāraṇā* (fixation). Fix your mind on *suśumna* (central nervous system). Now constantly and continuously initiate *dhyāna* (suggestion) from *suśumna* (central nervous system) to different parts of the body. Do not give suggestion in the beginning to all parts of the body, but select a particular part and then proceed to another part of the body systematically. For example, begin with the legs and relax them by your suggestion. Then abdomen, chest, arms, and head. Use *dhāraṇā* (fixation), *dhyāna* (suggestion), and *samādhi* (flowing of consciousness) in that order. In the beginning progress will be very slow. During the first few days, sometimes for a few months, you may not feel anything, but continue your practice daily and regularly, and eventually you will be able to relax your whole body within a moment and feel an ocean of supreme consciousness in and around you.

There are three classes of *pratyāhāra* (relaxation), according to degrees of relaxation:

1. State of *dhāraṇā:* This is called the very light state, or state of physical changes. In this state the student is not able to open his eyes. All voluntary muscles (hands, arms, legs, etc.) are relaxed and are in a sleeping state. The student is absolutely conscious of everything that is happening and, if he is in class, everything that is being taught by the teacher.
2. Intermediate State: This second state is the state of the individual mind and individual consciousness. The body and senses are under complete control of mental suggestion. The body and senses begin to sleep in a deeper state, deeper relaxation. The mind is full of light and consciousness is positively felt. It becomes the Self of the meditator. This is the state of *dhyāna* (suggestion), where all senses work relatively and the mind becomes free from the activities of sensory and motor organs; it enters the ocean of Universal Consciousness.

3. *Samādhi:* In this third state the body sleeps soundly. An operation can be carried out, even heart surgery might be performed, but there is no experience of pain. The body is completely in deepest sleep. There is no sleep like this sleep. We can only indicate that the body is completely under the command of the mind and the mind is submerged in the ocean of supreme consciousness. This is the deepest state. The mind is enlightened. In another state, truth is opened before him, but in this state he himself becomes truth. This is the state of *samprajñāt samādhi* (absolute enlightenment), where he identifies himself with supreme consciousness, supreme knowledge, supreme blessings, and supreme existence.

Practice daily and feel these states. They will come gradually to you. During the first few months it will take time and effort to achieve the first state, but when you have obtained the first state you will have tremendous confidence and enthusiasm for your practice of concentration; in time you will have all other states. Remember one word a million times: Practice —Practice—Practice.

There is another, a fourth state, called *turiya* (*asamprajñāta* or *nirvikalpaka samādhi*). This is the state where the student enters into that consciousness which is one-without-a-second. Here he sees the whole universe within himself, and vice versa, himself in the whole universe. This is *nirvāṇam.* This is the end of all practices. He obtains the true form of life. Here, books and scriptures cannot help him. One sees Self by the power of Self in the same way that, at dawn of day, all lights fail before the sun, and one sees the sun by the light of sun only.

Now you have come to the end of the second lesson. Study it, understand it, contemplate, concentrate according to it, before you go on to the next lesson.

3

SAMYAMAH AND YOGANIDRA—TRAYAMA EKATRA SAMYAMAH

Now you are familiar with the terms *dhāraṇā, dhyāna,* and *samādhi* (fixation, suggestion, and consciousness). After a few months of practice you will have sufficient will power to turn your body into complete *samādhi.* When fixation, suggestion, and consciousness operate together, they can turn the body into *samādhi* in a millionth of a second. This is like a waterfall of magnetic force in the field of individual consciousness. When the psychic electromagnetic current of fixation, suggestion, and consciousness steadily flow together like a mighty waterfall, it is called, technically, *saṃyamaḥ* (*sam,* complete; *yamah,* control of mental power).

Practice constantly and you will obtain *saṃyamaḥ.* At the state of *saṃyamaḥ,* you do not take time to control your mental and physical current. At your command the entire body, or any particular part, goes into sound sleep and consciousness is liberated and begins to submerge into the ocean of eternal existence, consciousness, and blessing.

Yoganidra is the technical form of Yoga. Yoga means concentration; *nidra* means sleep; that is, sleep resulting from complete concentration. When you use *saṃyamaḥ* for general or local concentration, respectively, a general or a local part of the body goes into what seems to be deep paralysis. In this state there is no sensation in any particular part. You cannot raise or move the entire body or any particular part of it. But do not be alarmed; this is not paralysis. It is a state of highest victory of mind over matter. This sleep is entirely different from other sleep, because you can summon it at your will and remove it at your will. If in this state even a heart operation were performed, you would not feel any pain. This is like a local anesthesia. In this state, pain, pressure, touch, temperature are out of awareness. When heat or cold, pain or pressure is applied to an organ, you cannot recognize or feel it. This *nidra* is due to your *saṃyamaḥ:* complete concentration. Therefore, it is called *yoganidra.* In *yoganidra* the body is sleeping soundly and the mind is awakening steadily.

Mind becomes the master of body and senses and not figuratively but practically exercises its mastery over senses and body. Just as under local or general anesthesia surgeons remove a diseased part of a body and restore health to the patient, so the student of Yoga under general or local anesthesia of *yoganidra* removes all mental and physical diseases that are transmigrating through innumerable incarnations and parental diseases inherited through the chromosomes of the generative cells; when all mental and physical diseases are eliminated, the purified mind begins to shine like the mighty sun after the disappearance of clouds.

Saṃyamah is a mighty power of mind. When it is awakened, *kuṇḍalinī* (potential power) is awakened. For your practice and to awaken your *kuṇḍalinī,* sit in a comfortable posture. Remember *saṃyamaḥ.* For example, select your arms first. Fix your attention on the whole arm and initiate suggestion in the following manner:

"Now I am going to relax my arm. I relax my arm. I relax my arms, I relax my arms." Repeat it constantly. Now send suggestion: "My arms are relaxing; they are relaxing; they are growing heavier; they are growing very heavy; although I wish to move them, to raise them, I cannot do so because they are completely relaxed by my eternal mind." Thus you repeat suggestion. One day you will see that your arms are really relaxed and you will begin to feel consciousness separate from your arm, and your arm is in *yoganidra.* Now you apply the same formula, process, and suggestion to another part of the body. Thus, in time you will be the master of your body. It is as easy as anything could be if you practice regularly. You will feel immeasurable peace and happiness because you have awakened the sleeping potential energy of the Self in yourself.

Any worthwhile achievement is impossible without practice, and nothing is impossible with practice. The men who became great Yogis and masters of mind were just like you are today. They started their practice of Yoga and gradually conquered death.

Now you come to the end of the third lesson. Before going on to the next lesson, study it, understand it, and apply it.

4

THE CITTAM: MIND, EGO, AND INTELLECT—THE LAWS OF THE MIND

Before entering into the practice of concentration, you have to understand the mind and the laws of the mind. To understand the mind, observe an infant, a child, and an adult fully developed mentally and physically. The infant tries to put everything into its mouth. It does not recognize the difference between subject and object. It sees everything as itself and wants to grasp everything and eat everything. It does not recognize the difference between good and bad. A growing child senses good as good and bad as bad, but in accordance with his environment. However, he tries to understand the difference between good and bad, subject and object. Sometimes he mistakes good for bad and bad for good, but he differentiates the two. A fully developed normal man should understand good as good and bad as bad, and their far-reaching influences for his development. He should have less doubt, and be equal to the judgment of things and of surroundings.

In the same way, that part of consciousness which is like an infant is called mind. This part of consciousness understands everything for itself. When it is developed, it becomes ego consciousness. It is now the principle of reality. That part of consciousness which understands real as real and unreal as unreal and uses reality to develop its personality and to dismiss unreality from life is called ego consciousness (the growing child). The intellectual consciousness is that part of consciousness which is the judicial branch of understanding, like a fully developed person. Ego consciousness is the executive branch, while intellectual consciousness or super ego is the judicial branch of it. It gives the final decisions for everything. While ego consciousness is the principle of reality, super ego is the principle of ultimate reality.

All three are working together. They are never separate. When these three work in the mental field, they create the world of animals; when they work in the field of ego consciousness, they create the human world; and when they operate in the world of super ego or intellect, they open heaven within the mind. Since they all work together in different planes, Yoga uses one technical term for them: *cittam* meaning the seat of *citti,* consciousness.

The term "mind" has widespread use, hence it is used for all three. Sometimes beginners feel confusion, but they should understand the meaning of mind according to sense and use. When we speak of the laws of the mind, we mean laws of the mind, ego, and super ego (*cittam*). We mean all three.

In order to practice Yoga and autosuggestion, it will be necessary to understand mind, ego, and intellect or *cittam* and their laws. As by the process of mental and physical development a baby is developed into a child and a child into an adult, so in the development of practice of Yoga the mind, transformed into ego consciousness or reality principle and ego consciousness, is further transformed into the ultimate reality principle or intuition. As a childish nature is controlled by young nature, and young habits are controlled by adult habits, so mental habits are controlled by ego and ego character is controlled by intellect and intuition.

Cittam is the arena of conflicting forces where war between divine and demon forces is constantly going on. The student of Yoga must control his demon forces and has to develop divine forces. This is the aim of Yoga. To check lower nature and develop higher nature is the process of meditation.

No one has been able to separate the parts of the mind, but for the purpose of Yoga—according to manifestation of consciousness—for all practical purposes, mind or *cittam* is divided into three levels:

1. Conscious mind: Example, waking state.

2. Subconscious mind: Example, dreaming state and sound sleep.
3. Superconscious mind: Example, concentration and *samādhi.*

There are a few other states, such as the unconscious and semiconscious, but all these are abnormal states of the mind and they are parts of the subconscious mind.

The conscious mind is the consciousness that is manifested through the proper functioning of the physical brain or cerebrum. It is manifested and developed according to the development of the brain and it perishes with the body. The subconscious mind is responsible for heart movement, circulation, digestion, respiration, creation and development of organs, etc. It works in the living body and it can work independently without the body and never perishes. Conscious mind is nothing but the by-product in the operating process of the subconscious mind and it cannot exist without the subconscious mind.

When through meditation, contemplation, and concentration psychic energy is transformed into higher energy it is called *superconscious mind.* This is a free state of consciousness, manifested only through *samādhi.* Otherwise, throughout their lives, people have only two states of mind: conscious and subconscious. Superconscious is the manifestation of the Universal Consciousness in *samādhi,* through complete concentration.

For beginners it is not necessary to discuss all the laws of the mind, but the mention of a few will aid the student in acquiring sufficient control of his conscious and subconscious mind to enter the superconscious state of mind through the power of suggestion:

1. The superconscious mind is that mind which manifests superconsciousness. Man can obtain this mind only through *samādhi.* In the state of superconscious mind, one perceives an infinite magnetic current around and within one's self. One sees inexpressible peace and happiness. In this state, all physical and mental diseases and other burdens are eliminated. One feels freedom within one's self. One obtains unbelievable powers. Nobody could describe the

boundary of the infinite. The aim of *samādhi* is to obtain this mind and this state.

2. The discharge of psychic energy through the *kuṇḍalinī* path or *suśumna* (central nervous system) manifests waking consciousness, and this state of mind is called conscious mind. It governs organs of actions and senses up to a certain extent, such as the voluntary muscles, organs, and functions of the body—the senses of taste, touch, smell, sight, hearing, etc.
3. The conscious mind operates from the breaking of one sleep to the beginning of another sleep.
4. The conscious mind tries to follow reality in life. although it faces great difficulties, sometimes calamity, to follow truth.
5. The conscious mind increases with proper training education, and good environment. It decreases without training and education and with unfavorable environment.
6. The conscious mind uses forces of induction and deduction; perception and inference; analysis and synthesis; logic and philosophy; science and art.
7. The conscious mind wishes to become master over both matter and spirit.
8. The conscious mind is the waking mind and the mind of activities. This is the mind of success and failure.
9. It is the mind through which you perform your daily work, and is a broadcasting station.
10. It has full freedom to select the divine or the demonic, and it has power to accept or reject any path, idea, proposition, or suggestion at its own disposal.
11. The conscious mind has limitless power, hence it performs every action.
12. The conscious mind cannot remember everything at the same time. Its past activities and experiences take the form of memory, which is stored up in the subconscious mind; hence its memory is limited and imperfect. It remembers according to the condition of the central nervous system. When the central nervous system is degenerated, it forgets everything, even its own individual name, children, family, city, country, etc.

13. The conscious mind is the cause of bondage and freedom of the Self. If it selects a material and lower way of life, the Self goes into bondage, and vice versa, if it selects the spiritual and higher way of life, it liberates the Self.
14. The conscious mind is the leading power and leader of all states and all minds.
15. The conscious mind can transform poison into nectar and nectar into poison; hell into heaven and heaven into hell; life into death and death into life; mortality into immortality and immortality into mortality. In short, it has the power and full freedom to become highest on the way to God and lowest toward the demonic.
16. The conscious mind constitutes the gross body (*sthūla śarīram.*)
17. The psychic energy discharged through *iḍa* and *pingala* (autonomic nervous system), which has its center in the *kuṇḍalinī* path, *suśumna* (central nervous system), constitutes the subconscious mind.
18. The subconscious is divided into three divisions: subtle, subtler, and the subtlest. The first two constitute *sūksma śarīram* (subtle body), and the last constitutes *suśupti śarīram* (causal body).
19. All involuntary functions of the body are governed by the subconscious mind, such as the involuntary muscles, organs, functions of the heart, lungs, digestive system, metabolism, kidneys, and the endocrine glands, etc.
20. The subconscious mind works constantly, in the waking state, dream, sound sleep, shock, coma, accident, etc.
21. In prolonged coma or anesthesia, the subconscious mind continues to act, and consequently the body continues to breathe and the heart continues to circulate blood. In short, all involuntary functions are in operation.
22. Unconscious mind has infinite power to alleviate life's pain and the suffering of the conscious mind. All pains, sufferings, and mental worries cease to operate. When the subconscious mind takes over and one is in this state, one is called unconscious.

23. The subconscious mind is the eternal storehouse of all memories, activities, and experiences. It projects them through conscious, waking, dream, and sound sleep states.

24. The subconscious mind has absolute control over all functions and sensations in the body.

25. Subconscious mind is amenable to all suggestions, whether they are mental, verbal, or environmental, if they are given properly.

26. Dream and sound sleep are the special modifications of the subconscious mind.

27. The subconscious mind will react according to intensity, amount, and degree of suggestion. If suggestions are strong and immediate, it will respond strongly and immediately. If they are in medium degree and mediate, it will respond in medium capacity and mediately. If they are weak, weaker, and weakest, the response will be weak, weaker, and weakest. If they are in a dormant state, it will register them in a dormant state and no action is taken.

28. The subconscious mind is without name, form, and personality, while the conscious mind has name, form, and personality. The subconscious mind works like God and does not demand any reward, while the conscious mind works like man and does not want to do anything without reward and remuneration.

29. When conscious and subconscious minds meet, they are transformed into the superconscious mind.

30. The superconscious mind has eternal existence, eternal knowledge, eternal consciousness, eternal peace, eternal happiness, eternal blessings, and eternal electromagnetic influence and control over all minds. It is the last law giving full freedom to the student of Yoga. Your success in Yoga depends upon the manifestation of the superconscious state of the mind. Remember: all states of the mind are relatively real, hence they are conditional, but the superconscious state is permanently real and therefore it is unconditional. When the superconscious state dawns on the firmament of the mind, all states disappear, as night disappears before the dawn of the day. Everybody, high or low, rich or poor, ignorant or wise, healthy

or sick, potentially has this state, but it is manifested fully only through *samādhi* (concentration). All states of the mind are dancing on this state. This is the fundamental substance for all states.

Now you come to the end of the fourth lesson.

The purpose of Yoga is to assist its students in the development of the superconscious state. We are concerned with practice, rather than theories without practice; physical and mental developments, rather than dry philosophy; simplicity rather than complexity. The laws and principles taught by Yoga are gaining momentum with great rapidity because these laws are in accordance with modern research and the investigations of science and psychology, and because Yoga avoids useless theory, which merely confuses the student of philosophy and science.

Yoga teachings are confined to the operation of the eternal laws of supreme nature and give no support to false speculation and abstractions.

5

RULES FOR PRACTICE OF YOGA

Before you learn the methods of Yoga, it is extremely important that you learn the manner of the Yogis. These simple rules are of the utmost importance:

1. Keep before the mind the fact that you have firmly decided to reform your life and to transform your conscious and subconscious mind into superconscious mind.
2. Enrich yourself with every possible truth and renounce untruth and prejudice as soon as possible.
3. Every mental and physical condition is in accordance with the judgment of supreme consciousness and supreme nature. The child may weep if an operation is needed but parents decide to do the operation to save the child. In the same way, you are unhappy and full of anxiety, but this operation on your mind is permitted by nature to save you from destruction. Even death is nothing but the greatest operation; after this operation, old age is removed and the Self is incarnated again as a child. Ponder over it and be free from all cares of body and mind.
4. An unhappy and restless mind cannot concentrate. Make every possible effort to make your mind happy and peaceful. The standard of admission in Yoga is a peaceful and happy mind.
5. Increase the atmosphere of expectancy and remove melancholy from the mind.

6. Believe in yourself and in your mind, and that you will obtain the supreme state.
7. If you fail to obtain some positive results in your practice, do not lose confidence. Owing to your inexperience, you are not yet able to recognize the positive higher changes in your mind. You may have the traditional habit of looking at the back of your mind.
8. Make it a habit to stand as a witness in every mental activity. Thus, you will save yourself from being the agency of mind and become the guide to your mind as an instructor. Don't play with your mind as if you were a servant and an agent. If you do so, you will face calamity.
9. Truth in speech, simplicity in manner, and firmness of mind are infallible divine instruments to certain success.
10. You must concentrate your mental waves with utter and complete confidence in yourself and in the nature in you and around you, which have manifested innumerable suns, stars, and planets.
11. Don't be nervous; a nervous attitude may interfere with your performance.
12. Know this: Mental and natural powers are looking to you to give you something that you have never seen before. They want to enrich you with divine and eternal powers. Eternal forces are serving you constantly, whether you know it or not. Before birth and after death, where no material things can go with you, these natural forces are serving you. Wherever you go, they are there before you.
13. Remember, you can do anything and everything that has been done by any great Yogi or Saint in human history. By your performance you can become a son of God, and by the highest performance you can become one with God. Nothing is impossible to the mind.
14. One wave of the mind is always skeptical of everything. Do not consider this wave as an ordinary one. Try to solve it in a right way through your instructor and practice; otherwise skepticism will wreck your performance. Here or hereafter there is no success

or happiness for the skeptical. Always, from the beginning of your practice, it will try to create doubt and suspicion in your practice, but after a few days of practice these mental waves will be the first to applaud your success in concentration. These mental waves of skepticism at first refuse to recognize anything. They recognize facts: nothing but facts. No philosophy, no religion, no gods or God is recognized by these waves. They recognize only direct experience. Therefore, to conquer these waves, practice constantly. They recognize your successful experimentation. When these waves perceive directly the eternal electromagnetic current of supreme consciousness, they recognize your feat and become your fast friend. When you have mastered your skeptical nature and obtained the right method of autosuggestion (*dhyāna*), you will have powerful mental waves in your favor. Now those waves which are weaker and still present in your mind cannot disturb you because you have seen the truth. Now you are not only the master of your mind, but you are going to become the master of all material minds.

15. Practice of Yoga will open the third eye in you, which is called "Yoga *dṛiṣṭi*," "*divya dṛiṣṭi*," or "divine eye."
16. Demand complete silence from your material mind and command it completely. When you achieve this control, nothing can disturb your practice.
17. Do your practice seriously. If you do it lightly, you may lose faith, confidence, and enthusiasm in yourself.
18. When you see any extraordinary vision, feel no fear; otherwise you may have a nervous breakdown, or you may harbor fear of ghosts or of death in your mind. No harm can befall you. Go into deepest experimentation. Place your body in a comfortable position and soon you will magnetize your body. Your mind will soon be enlightened.
19. There is one other peculiar disturbing wave of the mind: the wave of arrogance. In practice you obtain success, and success sometimes brings conceit, and conceit brings hypocrisy. Be careful. Do not harbor

this wave in your mind, as it may ruin you. You are not doing anything that has not been done previously by Yogis. It is not you but supreme consciousness and nature that want to present you before the world for the service of all living beings. Be careful not to become arrogant and conceited. Respect all more than yourself.

20. A proper and clear-cut suggestion is important to your mind. If you do not start distinct and powerful autosuggestion, your mind will start its own suggestion to you, and you will be governed by your mind. By powerful autosuggestion govern your mind, but do not let yourself be governed by your material mind.

Now you have finished this fifth lesson. Close your eyes and recall all the rules. Consider them. Read the lesson again, close your eyes, and remember it. Do this until you remember the lesson by heart.

Enrich yourself by the knowledge of anatomy, physiology, psychology, and other sciences to obtain the utmost success in the eternal science of Yoga.

Nothing is greater than self-knowledge. Make autosuggestion (*dhyāna*) a vital force in your concentration. Read it. Think of it. Practice it and feel it.

6

TRĀTAKAM: TRAINING THE GAZE

When fixation, suggestion, and sensation (*saṃyāmaḥ*—total concentration) are directed to the exterior surface of the body or to any external object, it is called *trāṭakam*. To obtain certain and earlier success, one should diligently follow the text or the teacher. Here I wish to point out some most important methods and rules for *trāṭakam* (concentration with open eyes):

A commanding *trāṭakam* (gaze) ranks in importance next to suggestion. To control mental waves and to check restlessness of the mind, a strong gaze is absolutely necessary. It is extremely necessary to obtain mastery in *pratyāhāra* and *yoganidra,* which will be taught later on in this course. Select a quiet private room for this practice. Classification is as follows:

1. Exterior surface of the body.

   a. Nasal gaze: Keep your eyes half closed, half open, and steadily gaze at the tip of the nose. Practice regularly in the morning and evening. When the eyes are tired or tearing, close them fully and meditate one minute in that state. When tiredness is removed, start your practice again. In the beginning you will feel different reactions, such as headache, giddiness, dizziness. Do not worry about them. These are reactions. They come and go. When you have any reaction, close your eyes and meditate on *anāhat nādam*—OM sound. Increase your practice gradually. Practice will strengthen your *trāṭakam*. In the beginning practice in five-minute periods. The nasal gaze (*trāṭakam*) will awaken your *kuṇḍalinī śakti,* which is in potential form in the *suśumna* (central nervous system). *Trāṭakam* will stimulate all centers in the brain by means of the cranial and spinal nerve centers, especially the optic and olfactory nerve centers, through association fibers. You will begin to perceive a wonderful smell around you and conquer all aches and pains in your head. A wonderful memory is the by-product of this practice. By this exercise you will soon be able to control the wandering waves of your mind. If you continue to practice the nasal gaze regularly for several months, you will be able to control mental and physical diseases and thus you will experience a perceptibly beneficial effect upon your previously unsteady mind.

CAUTION: The *nāsagra dṛiṣṭi* (nasal gaze) directly influences the whole central nervous system and peripheral nervous system through the olfactory nerves and optic nerves and through their association fibers, going to different nerve cells in the central nervous system. Therefore, this gaze should be practiced very slowly and cautiously. No one should undertake this practice without first consulting an expert instructor.

b. *Bhrumadhya dṛiṣṭi* (frontal gaze): Fix your power of attention at the center between the eyebrows. Turn your half-closed eyes toward the space between the eyebrows. Like the nasal gaze, the frontal gaze is a powerful exercise to control wandering thoughts and mind.

Comparison between nasal gaze and frontal gaze: In both gazes the central nervous system and the autonomic nervous system are awakened through different associations of cranial nerves, especially those nerves which innervate the nose, eyes, face, and neck. In the nasal gaze, fixation, suggestion, and consciousness or sensation are directed toward the tip of the nose and through it to the central nervous system, while in the frontal gaze they are directed to the space between the two eyebrows which is generally termed the "third eye" because it opens the eye of knowledge. In nasal gaze the upper half of the eyes is closed and lower half is open, while in frontal gaze the lower half is closed and upper half is open. You will become more familiar with the differences by your practice.

2. *Trāṭakam* on external objects: Select a picture of a perfect Yogi or respected teacher; or you can select some small, round object on the wall of your room if you do not know any liberated soul: a round object, a miniature, small round point, or zero. Think of the thing selected that it is the symbol of infinite nature, and by gazing at the symbol you are gazing at supreme consciousness and supreme nature. Place yourself in such a posture and position so that you may see this object easily: neither too far from it nor too near to it. Look at this object steadily. Practice constantly and regularly. Never gaze long enough to tire your eyes. Close your eyes and meditate in this state when you feel strain. After a few months of constant and regular practice you will increase your power to stare at this object almost indefinitely without strain, fatigue, and blinking.

   If, however, you find that you are not progressing or you are slow in achieving *trāṭakam* or you continue to feel some difficulty, such as strain, repeat the following process: With two fingers, the index and middle finger, placed gently on the eyelids, draw them closed. Hold them closed for a few seconds and send suggestions: "I relax my eyes; I relax my eyelids." Repeat this suggestion and you will begin to feel the sensation that strain, fatigue, and other difficulties are overpowered and the eyes are heavy in the sleeping state of *yoganidra*. This process will remove all your trouble. Practice *trāṭakam* to obtain will power. It is important to your future success in *pratyāhāra* and *samādhi*. In addition, it will produce a tremendous confidence in yourself and enthusiasm for practice.

3. *Trāṭakam* on a blue light: Place a bed lamp with a blue, very low voltage bulb at the head of your bed

or in other suitable place so that you can gaze easily. Now light the lamp and recline on the bed or an easy chair in the most comfortable posture. Place your arms and legs in an easy and relaxed position. No limb must be tense or rigid. Thrust out your legs and arms from your body. You can do this gaze by crossing the arms and legs separately or combinedly. Now gaze directly at the bulb in such a way that you do not blink your eyes. The light is directly overhead and you are peering intently at it. Your gaze must be steady, continuous, and constant. Concentrate fully on the bulb. Begin *pratyāhāra.* Relax your legs, abdomen, chest, neck, arms, and head; and feel that they are relaxing; they are relaxed; they are being magnetized, they are fully magnetized, and feel that the entire body is full of magnetic pulsation.

Gradually you will begin to lose all sense of feeling in your body. The muscles of the body will be anesthetized, the muscles of your mouth will sag. You will enter the world of *samprajñāta samādhi.* In a short time you will be unable to move your limbs and you will pass into deep Yoga *samādhi.* Never forget to repeat *dhāraṇā, dhyāna,* and *samādhi* (fixation, suggestion, and sensation). Repeat as long as you have no identity with supreme consciousness. As time goes on and you practice and become expert, you will develop will power to dominate your subconscious mind to the extent that it will obey your conscious commands.

NOTE: You can carry on the same practice by (1) putting the bulb behind you and gazing on the light of the bulb in your room, or (2) by putting the light behind an image or object.

Yoga is the system to instruct you in the various methods used to control the waves of the mind and to bring about *samādhi* (the state of supreme consciousness). These methods have been proved and perfected by innumerable students of Yoga through their experimentation.

Besides all methods taught to bring about *samādhi* and *yoganidra,* you must always be supremely sure and positive to command your mind through powerful suggestion. You must never say to yourself: "I am going to try to concentrate, I am going to try to control my mind, I am going to try to remove my difficulties." These are weak suggestions and may produce negative results; they introduce very great chances of failure, and raise doubt in your own capacity. Never use a negative statement.

Make suggestions in the following way, with absolute certainty: "I control my mind and all mental waves. I magnetize my whole body. I concentrate on supreme nature and supreme consciousness, which have eternal existence, knowledge, and peace, and which are my real nature." "I am immortal and the incarnation of righteousness. I now turn my whole body into the state of *yoganidra* for such and such time." A tremendous amount of suggestion, expectation, enthusiasm, and confidence is extremely necessary in yourself before starting nasal gaze and other Yoga practices.

The mental waves and nature look at you with great respect. Supreme nature is ever ready to bless you with eternal existence, knowledge, and peace.

Remember this formula:

> I will obtain the Ultimate Truth and Ultimate Reality, and the ultimate aim of my life in this world—whether my body may remain with me or it goes into pieces. My bones and flesh may go into complete annihilation or may remain with me; I shall obtain the True Form of the Universe. Through innumerable incarnations good results; I have obtained a human body. I will not lose this golden opportunity and will certainly obtain *samādhi* and the Real Form of Consciousness. Calamity may come or go, mountains may break on my head, but I will not leave my promise to obtain *nirvāṇam.*
> —Lord Buddha.

Comprehend this formula and you will conquer all calamities.

Now you have come to the end of the sixth lesson. Close the book. Put it away for a while and then reread it slowly until you know the lesson by heart.

7

PRATYĀHĀRA

You have already completed the introductory chapters of your course, and now you are ready for the advanced concentration. You will attain advanced concentration through *pratyāhāra.*

The withdrawal of energy and consciousness from the routine objective, operation of organs, and fixation of that energy and consciousness in the mind through *suśumna* (central nervous system) is called *pratyāhāra.* Thus, *pratyāhāra* has two main parts:

1. Withdrawal of energy and consciousness from the organs.
2. Union of withdrawn energy and consciousness with the central organ, mind, through *suśumna* (central nervous system).

These two systems of *pratyāhāra* operate simultaneously with *saṃyamaḥ* (fixation, suggestion, and sensation). Therefore, *pratyāhāra* is complementary to *saṃyamaḥ.* Without *pratyāhāra,* one cannot accomplish *saṃyamaḥ.*

Pratyāhāra has two applications in the body: (1) local application, and (2) general application.

According to these two applications of *pratyāhāra,* there are two classes of concentration:

1. Local concentration in local *pratyāhāra.*
2. General concentration in general *pratyāhāra.*

When *pratyāhāra* is directed locally to the arms, legs, trunk, neck, face, eyes, etc., it is called local because in that moment withdrawal of energy and consciousness is limited to that particular part of the body, and union of energy and consciousness with the central organ, mind, is achieved through that respective part of the central nervous system. Fixation, suggestion, and sensation (*saṃyamaḥ*), too, go together. The result is that that particular part is magnetized according to your command. When *pratyāhāra* is performed all over the body at the same time, it is called general *pratyāhāra,* because at this moment energy and consciousness are withdrawn from the whole body, all sensory and motor organs generally, and there is union of that energy and consciousness with the central organ, mind, through the whole central nervous system. However, for beginners general *pratyāhāra* and general concentration are difficult. They should first practice local concentration and local *pratyāhāra,* and this will finally lead to general *pratyāhāra* and general concentration.

The energy of the subconscious mind is widespread and constantly misused by the autonomic nervous system. Through innumerable incarnations we have given materialistic suggestions to our subconscious mind and now they are autonomic and out of our command. Thus, by our own mistakes and wrong suggestions, we have hypnotized ourselves in the limited compass of the body, although our real nature is eternal, omniscient, omnipotent, and omnipresent.

Pratyāhāra is the process of the perceptual mechanism by which you will be able to transfer power from the subconscious mind to conscious and superconscious mind, and remove the hypnotic influence of ignorance from the mind. Thus you will have energy and consciousness under your command, and use of that energy will be at your disposal. When you have energy and consciousness at your command, you will be able to remove all mental and physical diseases, as well as ignorance. When mental and physical diseases are checked and ignorance is removed from life, the eternal consciousness shines brilliantly in the superconscious field of the mind, like the sun shines in the sky when clouds disappear.

In the practice of *pratyāhāra,* you will begin to gain a clear understanding of the power of fixation, suggestion, sensation, and consciousness. The practice of *pratyāhāra* will develop your will power, and after you have already developed your will power to a certain extent, you will have more confidence in yourself.

Practice of Magnetic Sensation. The universe is full of magnetism. Mighty magnetic currents are passing in and around us; we live eternally in this magnetic ocean but beginners cannot perceive this truth. We mention here a few simple tests for beginners to examine magnetic sensation:

Sit in sunlight, gaze steadily, and see the constant shower of fine components of nature. After a short practice you will see small vibrating, shining bodies around you. See different types of lights in yourself and around you.

Sit in sunlight. Close your eyes, and whatever you see with closed eyes is one class of magnetic fluid.

Pass your hand before your eyes while they are closed, and you will note the shadow of your hand. You feel this because your optic nerve is sensitive to this magnetic fluid.

Raise your head with closed eyes toward the shining sun, and you will see the whole universe full of a red magnetic ocean. In this state now pass your hand between your closed eyes and the sun, and you will see a change in color to violet and blue.

Look toward the sun for a few seconds or toward any shining body and close your eyes suddenly. You will see a change in the magnetic ocean because your retina is reacting to chemical substances.

Sit in the sunshine and look toward the horizon. Gaze steadily and you will begin to see the reflection of light from every part of the earth and horizon. You will feel a tremendous thrilling sensation and immeasurable enjoyment. After a few months' practice, you will feel one eternal light in yourself and around you, giving life to every element of nature.

Sit in your room, or anywhere, and make these experiments, the first with open eyes and the second with closed eyes:

1. Open your eyes and see different movements of natural waves and atoms. After a few months' practice, you will see that your chamber is full of magnetic currents and magnetic lights.

2. Close your eyes and experiment with optic nerve sensation. You will see a dense darkness around you. After a while you will see that dense darkness is changing into light darkness, and light darkness into different lights. You will see unbelievable light around you.

Perform both of these experiments in every degree of light, that is to say, in daylight, at night, in darkness, in semidarkness, in lamplight, in sunlight, in moonlight, etc.

These tests are to awaken your mind and to open extrasensory channels. Do not be alarmed when you see the tremendous power of nature. She is your mother and will permit no harm to befall you. Do not be nervous. Nervousness is regarded as a weak phenomenon of the individual mind, but remember that when a person is nervous, his basic instincts are much sharper than normally. You have to use this increased sensitivity to develop your knowledge and will power, and when will power and understanding are increased, you will understand the exact nature of your mind and the world around you.

Remember this: It is an important fact that when you concentrate, meditate, gaze, or make other experiments, you must have ideas, words, and suggestions ready in your mind and on your tongue. The wordings, suggestions, and methods are important factors of Yogic concentration. By these and other important factors of *pratyāhāra,* you will be able to introduce your ideas smoothly to your subconscious mind, and after a few months' practice you will have confidence in yourself, and you will achieve a complete cooperation of your subconscious mind and nature.

Now you have come to the end of the seventh lesson. Read it through again so that you will have a clear understanding of the different stages of the magnetic ocean and *pratyāhāra.*

Each chapter is designed to help you build up, within yourself, the knowledge and power to become perfect in the practice of *samādhi.*

8

PRACTICE OF PRATYĀHĀRA THROUGH SEVEN CAKRAS

Local Pratyāhāra and Local Concentration. For the convenience of local *pratyāhāra* and concentration, the body is divided into seven zones. The classification and division are anatomic, physiologic, psychologic, and biologic, and every zone is controlled by a *cakra* (neurohormonal mechanism).

1. The first is the neurohormonal mechanism which controls, governs, and regulates the male and female generative organs. In Yoga, this *cakra* is called *mūlādhāra cakram* (mūla, first, main, chief; *ādhāra,* foundation, support, substratum). Through this path psychic energy is constantly discharged by the subconscious mind. Concentrate mental powers, withdraw the whole energy from the reproductive organs, and fix this energy to the lower part of *suśumna* (central nervous system). "I relax my reproductive organs. They are relaxing. They are under my command." Repeat it and feel that you have completely controlled them. This will give you mastery of sex control. Anger, lust, and greed are controlled by *pratyāhāra* on this *cakram.*
2. The second is *svādhiṣṭhāna cakram.* Both legs are controlled, governed, and nourished by this neurohormonal mechanism. It is the center of the lumbar region. "I relax my legs; they are relaxing; they are growing heavy, very heavy," etc. Repeat this formula three times. With proper fixation and suggestion feel

the sensations taking place through suggestion. The legs will be completely under your command. They will be as cold as ice; the temperature will be below freezing point, if you desire. Also, they will be as hot as fire, if you wish. They will be relaxed at your will. You will be able to remove all pains, aches, and diseases from your legs. If your legs were cut, you would not feel any pain. Feel magnetic pulsation, magnetic circulation, and magnetic vibration in both legs. After a few months' practice you will note that within a moment your legs respond as directed. Thus, you will have conquered any hidden diseases of your legs and they are completely under your control.

3. The third *cakram* is *maṇipūrá cakram*. It controls all abdominal organs. Its center is in *suśumna* (central nervous system) above the lumbar region. Fix your mental power on all organs in the abdomen. Send suggestion. First control diseases by your powerful suggestions. Feel magnetic current, magnetic pulsation and magnetic vibrations in the abdomen. Think that this magnetic current is removing all abdominal diseases hidden or prowling, and you will see that all the organs in your abdomen are supernormal and perfect in health. You will feel that your whole abdomen is full of magnetic current and pulsation, and you will feel a victorious enjoyment in all your organs in the abdomen.
4. The fourth *cakram* is *anāhata cakram* in the chest. Its center is in the central nervous system. Relax your chest; when it is relaxed you will feel that electricity is passing from the heart to every part of the body. Your whole body will be full of magnetic current and pulsation. Regulate your breathing for more rapid success. Nobody can describe the power of this *cakram*. Practice it and feel it.
5. The fifth *cakram* is *viśudha cakram*. It is in the neck. Through it, both arms and the parts below and above the neck are controlled. The neck is the crossroad and vital center of *pratyāhāra*. Start fixation and suggestion on the neck and feel the sensations that are going on through your practice. When the neck is relaxed you will feel that it is full of magnetic pulsation, current, and vibrations. Both arms will be as if com-

pletely anesthetized. Heat, cold, pain, pressure, touch, temperature are lost from the arms and now you can neither move them nor use them. They are completely paralyzed until you send them other suggestions. Practice it, feel it, and enjoy it.

6. The sixth *cakram* is *ājñā cakram*. This is the center of individual consciousness. Through *pratyāhāra*, individual consciousness is expanded into Universal Consciousness, and the whole body is relaxed completely; the whole body is full of mighty magnetic waves, pulsation, and vibration. You will not feel any pain, even if the heart were operated on and bones were removed from your body. Fix your power of attention between the two eyebrows, which is the center of the third eye, the eye of wisdom. Initiate suggestion to relax the whole body. For this *cakram* you must occupy a firm seat. Place your body in a suitable posture so that, in the deepest state, you will not have an accident and fall. This *cakram* will give you mastery over the whole body and you will join with supreme consciousness. No one can describe in human language this superhuman enjoyment. Concentrate on it, feel it, and enjoy it.
7. The seventh *cakram* is called *sahāsrāram*, which is the ultimate controller of all *cakras*. When the student reaches *sahāsrāram*, his individual entity disappears forever. He identifies himself with supreme consciousness. In this state he obtains *nirvāṇam*, which has eternal peace, eternal knowledge, and eternal blessings. Fix your power of attention on the whole *śirobrahman* (cerebrum), begin suggestion, and feel the sensation that the whole body is completely under your command.

General Suggestions for Local Pratyāhāra. Fixation, suggestion, and feeling of sensations are necessary for all *pratyāhāra*. Magnetic pulsation, circulation, and vibration are common to all *pratyāhāra*.

General Pratyāhāra and General Concentration. When the whole body goes into the state of *yoganidra*, the state of magnetism, in a moment, the state is called general *pratyāhāra*. This is the most advanced state and a student obtains it when he is first perfect in local *pratyāhāra*. In

I

SIDDHĀSANA

The posture is Siddhāsana, the easy meditative posture

other words, local *pratyāhāra* ends in general *pratyāhāra* and general concentration. In the advanced state you do not need to magnetize your limbs separately. By a single order, the whole body becomes magnetized. Thus, the practice of general *pratyāhāra* leads to the state of *samādhi.*

N O T E : If in the practice of local as well as of general *pratyāhāra* you are demagnetized, magnetize yourself in the same way. This time you will magnetize yourself sooner.

Now you have come to the end of the eighth lesson, which deals with the practice of local and general *pratyāhāra,* as well as with concentration.

Read it, understand it, think over it. Practice it and feel it.

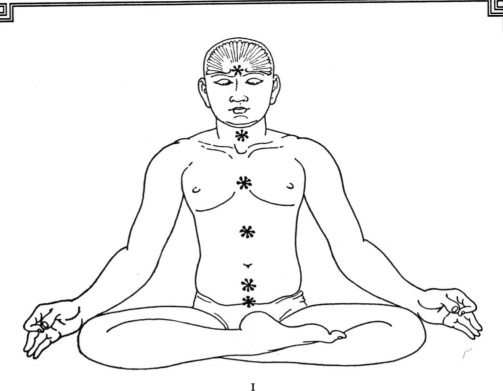

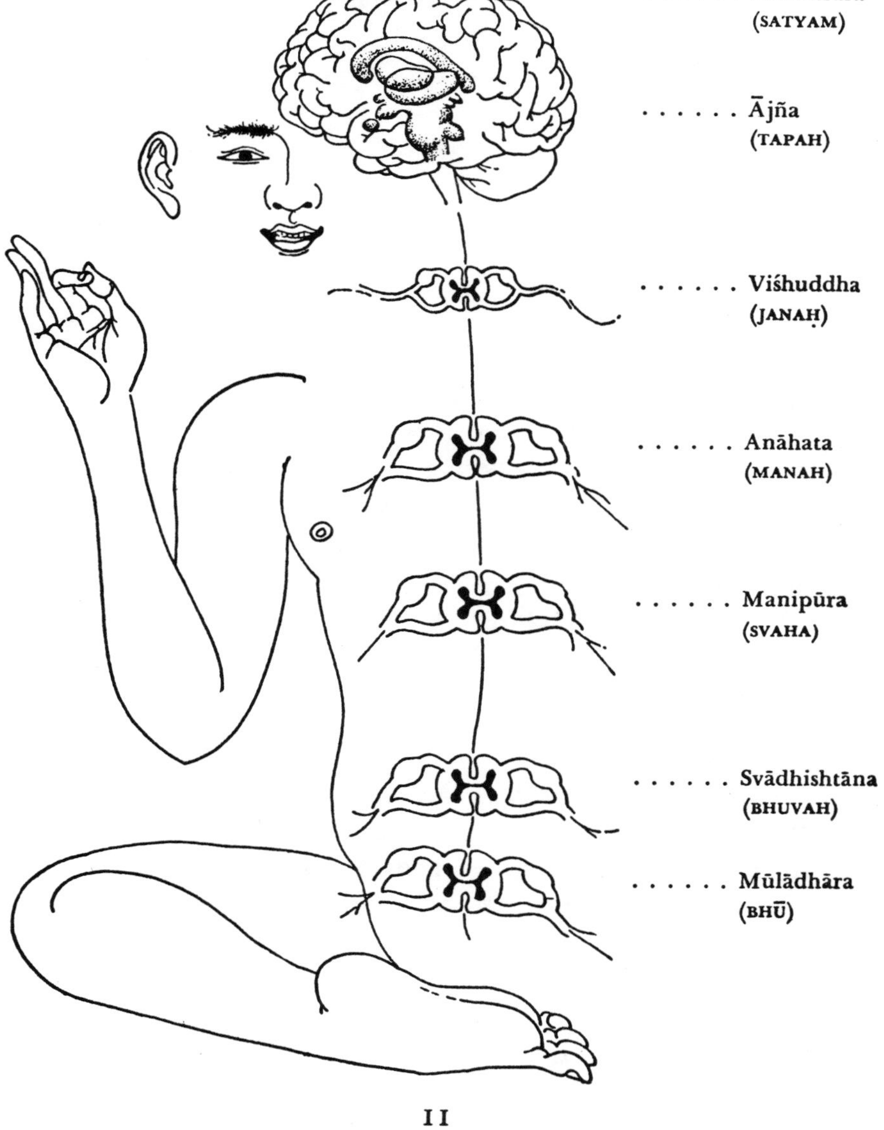

II

SEVEN CAKRAS

9

YOGANIDRA

Before proceeding with the next lesson, it will be well to learn the exact science of *yoganidra*. A brief introduction to *yoganidra* has already been given in preceding chapters. Now you will be able to understand it more fully. Only through a thorough knowledge of *yoganidra* will you be able to conquer your difficulties and imperfections, and you will be a *siddha* Yogi; that is to say, have command over nature. Any person can become a Yogi, but there is a great difference between a *siddha* Yogi and a Yogi. By obtaining mastery over *yoganidra,* even an ordinary Yogi may become a *siddha* Yogi.

Yoganidra is a state of magnetism. Through *dhāraṇā, dhyāna,* and *samādhi* the body, senses, and material mind are magnetized. The whole body is completely anesthetized. Even if the heart is operated on and bones are removed from the body, a student of *yoganidra* does not feel any kind of pain in the state of *yoganidra. Yoganidra* does not indicate only the sleep due to Yoga, but it is a technical term of Yoga that includes innumerable phenomena and manifestations of Yoga.

To magnetize the body, first you have to understand how to use fixation, suggestion, and sensation, and how to use the proper pause for time. First fix your power of attention for local or general *yoganidra;* then initiate powerful suggestion, and then pause to feel sensation of that suggestion which you have already given. If you give suggestion constantly and do not allow for a pause to feel the result of your suggestion, you cannot obtain the expected result of your suggestion.

I assure you that you will become a *siddha* Yogi if you will study what I teach you. Keep practicing. It is as simple to become a *siddha* Yogi as it is to swim in water. Practice *dhāraṇā, dhyāna,* and *samādhi* and success will come to you rapidly.

When you begin to practice Yoga and *samādhi* and begin to demonstrate Yoga performance as a student of Yoga, many people, and perhaps first your own family and friends, will ask you the question: "What is Yoga? What is *samādhi* and what is *yoganidra*?" and the like. To answer these questions intelligently, you have to understand the following definitions: Yoga is *kaivalyam;* that is to say, the obtaining of that highest state, which is one-without-a-second. *Samprajñāta samādhi* is the state of union of individual consciousness and Universal Consciousness. *Asamprajñāta samādhi* is the state of identification of individual consciousness with Universal Consciousness. *Yoganidra* is the state in which the whole universal magnetic ocean comes under your command.

In the individual plane, your body, senses, and mind are magnetized and are completely under your command.

In the state of *yoganidra,* the whole body is magnetized and it becomes full of electromagnetic pulsation, vibration, and concentration. With these phenomena, the body becomes painless, respiration becomes occasional, the heart movement is sometimes rapid and sometimes very slow, according to the stimulation or depression of the cardiac center in the medulla oblongata (*suśumna śiśakam*). Anesthesia is manifested in different degrees, according to the state of *yoganidra.* It is from superficial to the deepest state, from local to general. There are marked cardiomuscular changes. Circulation of the blood becomes more effective. Every particle of the body pulses with blood, electricity, and magnetism. In the advanced state, the student begins to feel the whole atmosphere and universe pulsating and vibrating with his pulsation and vibration.

All physical and mental diseases are removed by the state of *yoganidra,* which is the greatest anesthesia when you are your own surgeon to operate on your material mind and to remove it from the body. *Yoganidra* makes you an engineer to construct a bridge between physics and metaphysics, to cross the ocean of materialism.

Beginners fall asleep when they start meditation. This is the first manifestation of *yoganidra.* In the advanced state, it begins its influence over the body with yawning.

Yoganidra is induced physiologically by repeated stimulation of postures and reflexes; psychologically by *dhāraṇā, dhyāna,* and *samādhi.*

There are a few other manifestations of *yoganidra,* such as the lethargic, cataleptic, and somnambulistic states. These manifestations will come to you, according to the degrees of *yoganidra:*

1. First state of *yoganidra:* The body becomes numb and superficial sensation of pain, pressure, touch, and temperature is lost. In the first stage the symptoms are very light. There is relaxation, gradual closing of the eyes, fluttering of the eyelids, torpidity of the limbs, lassitude in eyes, anesthesia in the lower legs and feet, lower arms and hands, inability to raise or move arms and legs. In the first stage of *yoganidra,* all superficial sensations are lost, but the individual is absolutely conscious of everything that is being done and said. This is the state of semiconsciousness, the first degree of magnetism.
2. Second state: All physical sensations, deep or superficial, are lost, and the body is magnetized. In the second stage of *yoganidra,* the body, senses, and mind become partially under control. There is a partial anesthesia of the whole body and complete anesthesia of all limbs. The body is magnetized in second degree. One sees a variety of visions.
3. Third state: The body is fully magnetized and becomes full of pulsation, blood circulation, and electrical discharges. The whole atmosphere and universe become full of pulsation with this pulsation. This is the state of *samprajñāta samādhi.* In the third degree of anesthesia, the body is magnetized in the third degree, which is the last stage of individual magnetism. Temporary magnetism of the whole atmosphere is obtained, and also constant and regular visions of the Supreme. This is the state of union of individual consciousness with supreme consciousness. The material form of individual existence is united with Universal Matter, and the conscious part of indi-

vidual existence is united with Universal Consciousness. This is the state of godlikeness. According to the Gita, for the world He is sleeping, and for Him the world is sleeping. The material structure of the body is fully magnetized, and the mind is awakened and Enlightened. This is the state that is technically termed *samprajñāta samādhi* or *savikalpaka samādhi.*

4. Fourth state: The state of complete freedom from abstract bondage; the student feels identity with supreme consciousness, and nature is fully magnetized and becomes his body. In the fourth state of *yoganidra,* man is liberated from all bondages of the body. He obtains full freedom. Now the state of union is extended into the state of identity. He identifies the whole universe with himself, and himself with the whole universe. He obtains the state which is called *kaivalyam;* that is to say, that highest state of *nirvāṇam* which is one-without-a-second. Universal Nature is his body, and Universal Consciousness is his Self. He becomes the Self of all selves. No one can describe this state by tongue or pen. This is only an indication. Enter into that state and feel it! At this point the Yogi conquers entire nature.

General evidences of yoganidra:

1. A gradual closing of the eyes or motionlessness of the eyes.
2. Half closing of the eyes or quivering of the eyelids.
3. Complete relaxation or rigidity and stiffness of the limbs and other organs.
4. Temporary paralysis of the limbs and body.
5. The face may appear flushed.
6. Sometimes the teeth chatter.
7. Redness and sensation of heat or cold in different parts of the body.
8. Tears in one or both eyes.
9. Lightning around the body and in the body when eyes are closed.
10. Passing of electricity and electric currents in the body.
11. Jerking of body.
12. Different unusual phenomena that resemble delusions, illusions, and hallucinations.

13. Local anesthesia or general anesthesia.
14. Analgesia: loss of the sense of pain; indifference to painful stimuli.
15. Loss of body consciousness. In the beginning, there is loss of body consciousness locally; that is to say, sometimes the student feels that he has no head, no arms, no legs, etc., or sometimes he feels a disorientation of the body, as if the head, arms, and legs were somewhere else, etc.
16. Subjective or objective moving sensation. He feels that the head is moving or the atmosphere is moving around him.
17. Yawning.
18. Stretching of limbs.
19. Sleepiness or sleeplessness.
20. Power of intuition is increased.

NOTE: These are a few evidences of *yoganidra,* which are mentioned here to encourage the student to practice. It is not necessary that one must feel them all, or feel them chronologically. There are innumerable signs and evidences of *yoganidra.* When you have developed your intuition through concentration, you will recognize them. Books cannot guide you fully. The whole universe is a mass of concentrated energy. Therefore, it is in the state of *yoganidra.*

Now you have come to the end of the ninth lesson. Read it; close your eyes; remember it and ponder over it. Practice it and you will be able to create the state of *yoganidra* in yourself and in others.

10

METHODS FOR CREATING THE STATE OF YOGANIDRA

There are two methods of *saṃyamaḥ* (fixation, suggestion, and sensation) employed by Yogis to induce the state of *yoganidra:*

1. The Positive Method. (Active)
2. The Negative Method. (Passive)

THE POSITIVE METHOD

In the positive method we use the infinite power of OM sound to magnetize the whole body and the universe. You use the seven *cakras* for the positive method. First think of the positive nature of supreme consciousness and supreme nature. Innumerable suns and solar systems are manifested by this primordial principle. It is manifested in us in the form of *anāhata śabda* or *śabda brahman.* Divide your mind into three parts. The first part must be engaged in *anāhata nāda* (source of silence), the second part must be busy in magnetizing the body and senses locally and generally and the third part must examine the result of the whole process. Thus, with the help of *pratyāhāra* and *saṃyamaḥ,* relax all your organs: start from the legs and go to the abdomen, chest, neck, and arms; the third eye (the point between the eyebrows); and *sahasrāram* (cerebrum), respectively. Feel the sensation of blood circulation, pulsation, electromagnetic pulsation in every organ locally and in the whole body generally. After a few months' practice you will be expert in the positive method to induce *yoganidra.* When you can induce *yoganidra,* you will control all mental and physical diseases and be at one with supreme nature and supreme consciousness.

THE NEGATIVE METHOD

In the negative method you must forget your body and the huge external universe around you. You must remember only the virtues of the Self; that is to say, supreme consciousness. An ocean of consciousness will begin to flow around you and within you, and you will see that your body and the whole universe are melting in that infinite ocean. In this state you will see but one eternal principle, which is without name and without form, which has infinite power and infinite electromagnetic attraction for your body, the universe, and all of nature, and which has eternal consciousness, existence, knowledge, peace, and happiness.

This is the supreme state of *samādhi* and *yoganidra.* All of nature and the entire universe are transferred into the supreme state, which is one-without-a-second, and which is the subject of supreme *samādhi* and supreme *yoganidra.* No one can describe it.

Thus, you have two states to induce *yoganidra.* You will understand the second method when you are expert in the first method. The first method is one of compulsion and command and is indicated for rapid induction of *yoganidra* and *samādhi,* and controls the restless waves of the mind. The senses and body become motionless, sensationless, and they are magnetized by consciousness. The body becomes full of pulsation and electromagnetic current. All senses become co-operative and alert.

The second method is the method of identification of individual matter and consciousness with universal matter and consciousness. This is the state of perfect freedom. You can perform this method when you have already accomplished the first one. When, through the first method, all mental and physical diseases are controlled and all *karmas* are conquered, the Yogi obtains the second method. When the body is diseased, senses are irritated, and mind is restless, no one can perform the second method. How can one forget the body when it is already congested with mental and physical worries? First conquer your physical and mental worries by the first method, and when your mind is happy, senses are calm and the body is strong, enter into the second method and enlighten your mind.

You have to remember at least two constant factors in all methods:

1. According to the situation, apply some strong way to fix and maintain the power of attention over a period of time.
2. Apply firm *saṃyamaḥ* (fixation, suggestion, and sensation) through *pratyāhāra* for a period of time to create the state of *yoganidra.*

It is impossible to handle all mental waves and all problems by the same technique. Therefore, you must know different techniques and different solutions for your problems. Each problem and each mental wave must be regarded as an individual entity, presenting entirely different natures among themselves. After long practice you will know which method and which solution is the most suitable and favorable for you.

You should use a persuasive method when the mental waves are gentle and noble.

Now you have come to the end of the tenth lesson. Reread it and understand it. Put the book aside for a while, close your eyes, and meditate on it. Thus, you learn to control your mind and the mental waves that were beyond your control.

NOTE: In the positive way of meditation there are five planes of consciousness, while the negative way leads the aspirant to ultimate reality which is one-without-a-second and which is beyond the five planes.

I. PHYSICAL PLANE *(Annamaya Śarīram)*
II. ELECTRO-MAGNETIC PLANE *(Prānamaya Śarīram)*
III. PSYCHIC PLANE *(Manomaya Śarīram)*
IV. PLANE OF REVELATION *(Vijñānamaya Śarīram)*
V. PLANE OF ETERNAL EXISTENCE, ETERNAL CONCIOUSNESS AND ETERNAL BLISS *(Satchidānanadamaya Śarīram)*

Then there is one other state of consciousness beyond these five states, which is obtained only by the negative method of meditation by merging the previous states into the later ones successively, and lastly the fifth into the sixth, the plane of *Brahman.*

Technique.

1 Relaxation of the body and the mind

a. Removal of all tension and effort from the body

b. Renunciation of all undue material intentions of the mind.

2 Concentration of self-consciousness on *nādam*.

I. PHYSICAL PLANE. Concentrate on *nādam,* relax entire body. Relax skin, muscles, bones, organs, extremities; renounce all material desires and concentrate self-consciousness on *suśumna* (central nervous system). Start *saṃyamaḥ*. The entire body is relaxed. It is motionless. *Nādam* is increasing more and more. In a few months' practice you will find it easy to relax completely and feel the entire universe vibrating in the ocean of *nādam.*

II. ELECTRO-MAGNETIC PLANE. Go beyond the first stage and feel that the entire body is full of *prāṇa-spandanam* (electro-magnetic pulsation). First feel electro-magnetic current rhythmically pulsating in the entire body and then feel that the entire atmosphere is filled with this pulsation and, lastly, feel it in the entire universe. In a few months' practice you will be able to forget your physical consciousness and you will feel your body as a wonderful and eternal electromagnetic detector. This plane will open a tremendous and stupendous power of nature in you and around you.

III. PSYCHIC PLANE. After accomplishing the electro-magnetic field of nature, you will reach the motionless ocean of eternal electricity. This is not material electricity, but a very subtle electricity. Yogis call it psychic electricity. By experience you will know the penetrating power of the eternal mind.

IV. PLANE OF REVELATION. When you reach this state the meaning of manifested universe will be opened to you directly. You will perceive revelation of truth and world scriptures in your mind. You will understand the real significance and relation of the entire universe and the relation of the organic and inorganic world, as well as evolution, preservation and involution of both.

V. THE PLANE OF ETERNAL EXISTENCE, KNOWLEDGE AND BLISS is the plane of Supreme Consciousness. This state is the master of all. This is the knower of all; this is the inner controller; this is the source of all; this is the beginning and the end of all organic and inorganic worlds.

Up to the fifth state we recognize *Brahman* through expressions and symbolism which are presented to our consciousness by Supreme Nature. But the attainment of *Brahman* by the light of *Brahman* is called *nirvāṇam* and is beyond the five planes. It is called *Brahman* in Vedānt, *nirvāṇam* in Buddhism, and *nādam* and *praṇavam* in Yoga philosophy.

When all these states are mastered the aspirant realizes *Brahman* with the light of *Brahman,* as we see the sun with the light of the sun only. Successively accomplishing and mastering the later state, identity with the previous one is removed. This successive discovery leads to the final, the fundamental principle of the universe.

In the process of reaching up to *Brahman* all material coverings are removed from the self and reality is realized. It is called discovery and the aspirant applies the discovered principle to his practical life. Then it is called invention.

Once the later state is realized the notion of identity with the previous state is automatically rejected. This process of super-imposition and rejection *(adhyāropa* and *aphavāda)* is going on up to the final state of *Brahman,* and when it is realized all the five previous states are rejected, and the aspirant is established in the state of pure *Brahman.* This state is beyond all states and beyond all description. However, it is sometimes described negatively: It is not that which cognizes the internal object; not that which cognizes the external object; not that which cognizes both of them; not a mass of cognition, not cognitive, not non-cognitive. It is unseen by the physical eye; it is incapable of being spoken of; it is ungraspable, beyond all distinctive marks of all five planes of natural consciousness, unthinkable and unnamable. It is the essence of all four planes. It is the foundation of all evolution, preservation and annihilation of the universe. It is beyond distinction of subject and object and yet it is above and not below this distinction. It is not theism nor antitheism but supertheism. It is *Brahman* and it is *nirvāṇam.* It is one-without-a-second, and it is to be known and identified for final liberation.

From the empirical point of view there are three divisions of consciousness:

1 The waking state
2 The dreaming state
3 The state of sound sleep and all other unconscious states: coma, swoon, delirium, etc.

There is one other state of consciousness which is beyond these three. It is fourth in number and therefore is called *turiya. Turiya* is a figurative term. Actually it is not fourth in number. It penetrates all three empirical states and it is beyond them. *Turiya* is described above as the state beyond the fifth.

11

COMBINED POWER OF TRĀTAKAM

You are already familiar with *trāṭakam* and its significance (steady gaze). In this chapter you will learn the combined practice of *trāṭakam* with other practices. Combined practice produces combined power. Thus, you will have unbelievable forces of Nature with you. The following are a few important combined practices which are given for your convenience. You can establish additional ones if you believe that you will be able to handle them all:

1. *Trātakam* with nasal gaze (tip of the nose).
2. *Trātakam* with nasal gaze (bridge of the nose).
3. *Trātakam* with frontal gaze (root of the nose). That is, the third eye, the point between the eyebrows.
4. *Trātakam* with *mūlādhāra cakram,* to control lower desires, sex control.
5. *Trātakam* with *svādhiṣṭhāna cakram,* to control and magnetize the legs.
6. *Trātakam* with *maṇipūra cakram,* to remove all abdominal and metabolic defects and fill them with strong, healthy vibrations.
7. *Trātakam* with *anāhata cakram,* to feel pulsation and electromagnetic circulation in the whole body through the heart and chest.
8. *Trātakam* with *viśudhā cakram* to magnetize the neck and arms.
9. *Trātakam* with *ājñā cakram* (third eye) to feel unity of individual consciousness with supreme consciousness.
10. *Trātakam* with *sahasrāram śirobrahman* (cerebrum),

to feel identity with supreme consciousness.

11. *Trāṭakam* with room atmosphere to feel different natural lights and mental waves.
12. *Trāṭakam* with the horizon in sunshine to see the tremendous power of the sun and radiating and reflecting light and life from the sun to the earth.
13. *Trāṭakam* with full moon, to further awaken the mind.
14. *Trāṭakam* with books, to read them with electromagnetic force, without movement of the body.
15. *Trāṭakam* with *anáhata nádam,* OM or *Brahman,* to hear the eternal music of the universe.
16. *Trāṭakam* with interlaced fingers.
17. *Trāṭakam* with crossed ankles.
18. *Trāṭakam* with expanded arms.
19. *Trāṭakam* with standing posture and hanging arms.
20. *Trāṭakam* with any posture that the student feels suitable for himself.

General introduction to all combined trāṭakam. In all *trāṭakam,* power of attention is in two divisions:

1. The doer or agent.
2. The witness.

First, you open your eyes and gaze steadily at the part of your body which you have selected. Start with *pratyāhāra,* fixation, suggestion, and recording of sensations. The second part must be entirely as a witness to observe the result of the experiment and, if necessary, to help the first part in time. You can also apply this classification for other meditation.

Each *trāṭakam* has its own significance. You should practice them all, one by one. After a few months' practice you will have the power to express *trāṭakam* on your entire body. Through *trāṭakam* you will be the master of any and every organ. The organ will obey you according to your command. If you wish to transform it into the state of sound sleep, it will sleep; if you want to paralyze that organ temporarily, it will do so; if you want to magnetize and fill it with electromagnetic pulsation, it will do so. In short, whatever command you give to your body will be carried out immediately.

This is the end of the eleventh lesson. Close your eyes

and close your book; make a complete picture of all *trāṭakam* in your mind. Think of their significance. They give mastery over the body, senses, and the mind. If you have forgotten these twenty formulas of *trāṭakam,* reread them again until you have memorized them.

Meditate on these twenty formulas of *trāṭakam,* and when ready, begin your practice with one at a time. Do not practice all at the same time. When you are more experienced, you will be able to do so. Develop a working knowledge of anatomy and physiology in order to obtain more rapid success. Do not relate your success or experience to anyone who is not doing *trāṭakam,* as you might be misguided. If you have any questions, ask your teacher or an expert. You will obtain success according to your practice, if you practice seriously and faithfully.

12

TECHNIQUES TO MAGNETIZE THE BODY

As a student of Yoga, you will be obliged to adopt different techniques with different types of mental waves, and it is important that you know all of them. Every known and proved method of magnetism for *samādhi* will be taught to you in this course. These methods are used successfully today by innumerable students of Yoga, and you will also follow them easily. To become a successful and perfect Yogi, you should utilize every opportunity to experiment and to practice the science of Yoga. The methods should be learned one at a time; complete each before the next technique is taken up.

You are now ready to begin your first lesson on magnetizing your body, senses, and mind. This method is known by two names:

1. Local Magnetism.
2. General Magnetism.

When a particular part of the body is magnetized, this is called local magnetism; when the entire body is magnetized in universal magnetism, the term is general magnetism. The aim of local and general magnetism is to obtain universal magnetism. For this purpose you must achieve the following:

1. A working knowledge of anatomy, physiology, and psychology.
2. A perfect study of the circulatory system, the central nervous system, and the peripheral nervous system.

3. Understand the structure of the heart, its systolic and diastolic movements, and the blood vessels.
4. Complete relaxation of any particular part, or the entire body.
   a. When any particular part or the entire body is relaxed, you will begin to feel pulsation of the heart.
   b. Heart movement will increase with your psychic power.
   c. You will feel the whole body full of electrical discharges.
   d. After a few months of practice you will feel electromagnetic attraction in your body.
   e. You will feel that your whole body is full of electromagnetic attraction.
   f. Lastly, you will lose completely the sensation of your body, and feel that an ocean of magnetism and consciousness is flowing around you and within you. This is the state of universal magnetism.

The process is as follows:

Place your body in a comfortable posture.

Relax your body completely.

Repeat firmly *saṃyamah* (fixation, suggestion, and sensation).

By *pratyāhāra* (withdrawal of energy), take charge of consciousness and energy at your disposal.

When the body is relaxed, feel pulsation and electromagnetic attraction in the entire body.

Feel identity with supreme consciousness and *nādam*.

Forget completely the relation and union of the body at time of practice.

Your mind should register different sensations of nerve currents going on at the time of practice.

Remember the nature of the Self, which has eternal consciousness, existence, knowledge, peace, and bliss.

If lower desires come to your mind, check them

immediately.

NOTE: If, in spite of all these efforts and precautions, your body does not respond, repeat the above mentioned technique. The next time you will require less time to magnetize your body. Be quiet in your actions. Show no nervousness. Concentrate your mental power and physical forces upon what you are doing. Be firm of will and you cannot fail. When your body is magnetized, send the strong suggestion: "My body is completely magnetized. I cannot raise or move any part of the body in any direction because it is fully controlled and magnetized by my eternal mind." If the material mind moves any part of your body in any direction against your desire, check it by your eternal mind again. Remember that the eternal mind is greater than the material mind. You will feel that your body is really magnetized, and your material mind cannot move it now without your permission. When your time of practice is over, send your psychic force again to the entire body, through the nerves and vessels, and you will note that your body is strong, weakness is removed, and your mind is enlightened.

This is the end of the twelfth lesson. Read it; understand it. Practice, Practice, and Practice!

13

GROUP RELAXATION AND GROUP MAGNETISM

Group relaxation and group magnetism depend upon two principal conditions:

1. Ability of the teacher.
2. Co-operation and ability of the student or the group.

The percentage of relaxation and magnetism is in accordance with these two facts. If both conditions are 100 per cent perfect, the result will also be 100 per cent. It is always in accordance with the degree and proportion of both. Relaxation and magnetism are according to the ratio of the performance. The process is as follows:

You are all assembled to learn Yoga, meditation, concentration, and relaxation. Many persons come, not to learn, but to observe as visitors because they have some fear in their minds. However, they too have love for meditation, and curiosity to know something about Yoga.

First ask at your meeting, How many are visitors and how many are learners? Give an opportunity to all according to their readiness. Today's visitor may be tomorrow's learner. Do not compel visitors to become learners. Let them decide for themselves. Do not ask as to the results of your performance from visitors who were not ready to follow your orders. Ask those who were co-operative and ready for your instructions.

Begin with learners as follows: "Now you are ready for concentration. Be ready for *pratyāhāra* (withdrawal of energy and consciousness from different parts of the body), according to instruction. Place your body in a comfortable position. (If they cannot achieve *padmāsana,* the lotus posture, let them sit up straight in a chair.) Put your feet flat on the floor. Put your hands on your knees. Close your eyes. With great care and attention listen to me. Lead your mind from darkness to light. Lead your mind from lower existence to higher existence. Lead your mind from death, disease, and suffering to immortality. Lead your mind from unreal life to real life. Relax your entire body. Repeat *saṃyamaḥ* (fixation, suggestion, and sensation) mentally. I relax my entire body. My entire body is relaxing. Feel the pulsation of the heart in every part of the body. With great care and great attention feel pulsation in the chest. Inhale and hold your breath. With every pulsation, the heart is sending life, energy, and nourishment to every part of the body. With every pulsation, the entire body is being magnetized; every part is relaxing and the mind is awakening. Exhale." Repeat this formula mentally and you will feel that your whole body is relaxed and magnetized. "The entire body is filled with electromagnetic pulsation. OM sound—*anāhata nādam*—is increased. A great ocean of consciousness is flowing around you and within you. A great ocean of magnetism has attracted your entire body into universal magnetism. Now the force of magnetism is increasing and you have completely lost consciousness of your body. You have identity with supreme nature and supreme consciousness. The supreme consciousness, supreme nature, which has manifested innumerable stars, suns, moons, and planets is manifested in yourself and around you. Supreme consciousness is your nature. By ignorance you had superimposed the limitation and connection of the body on yourself. Now this limitation and connection of the body is over and you are in the ocean of Supreme consciousness. Supreme consciousness, supreme *Brahman,* is your Self. Now you are in your native land. Now you do not know where your body is. The entire universe is in you and you are in the entire universe. Innumerable suns, stars, and planets are moving in you. Feel it, enjoy your real life." Complete silence.

By repeating this formula, you will see that the learners are relaxed and magnetized, and the visitors sense some of the enjoyment of life as they participate in this Yoga performance; also they are experiencing an answer to their

CARDIAC CYCLE

This plate shows Lesser Circulation through lungs and Greater Circulation throughout the body. In higher meditation this represents electromagnetic pulsation in the individual body and in the atmosphere around the body. Consequently it leads the meditator from the individual electromagnetic field to the universal electromagnetic field. The meditator feels everywhere magnetic pulsation and forgets consciousness of his body.

1. Lesser Circulation, pulsation through chest
2. Greater Circulation
   - A. pulsation through arm and head
   - B. pulsation through liver
   - C. pulsation through intestines
   - D. pulsation through kidneys
   - E. pulsation through intestines

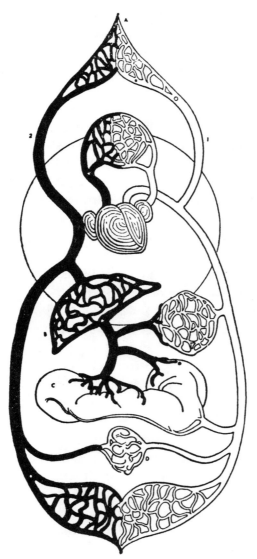

curiosity. Now they may be ready to learn Yoga. If some learners are not obtaining the expected results, owing to their physical and mental difficulties, do not be alarmed, because by repeating this formula they will conquer these obstructions and will obtain the expected results sooner or later. First, they will relax their bodies quickly and deeply. In the advanced state, the student will feel that with every pulsation of the heart his body is being magnetized and consciousness is awakening.

When the audience is relaxed and has lost its feeling of the body, and has identity with supreme *brahman,* begin chanting OM and other heavenly prayers. Compose your own prayers and chant them. If you cannot do so, repeat some good prayer. Do not chant an ordinary prayer and do not pray for selfish desires.

Pray for the welfare of the world. Every living being should be free from disease and sufferings; they should all be happy; all should enjoy identity with supreme *brahman* and none should be unhappy. "I do not want a kingdom. I want happiness for all. I do not want only my liberation. I want liberation for all. I do not want to remove pain and sufferings only from my body, but from all. The seasons, atmosphere, days, nights, years, planets, suns, moons, stars, oceans, rivers—all should be happy and mutually useful. OM, Peace, Peace, Peace."

Now you have come to the end of the thirteenth lesson. Read it, understand it, and practice it. OM.

14

POSTOPERATIVE AND POSTMEDITATIVE SUGGESTIONS

In this lesson we shall take up the very important subject of the result of meditation and concentration. This is the most amazing subject of Yoga. As a result of meditation, a crow is transformed into a swan; a sinner becomes a saint; the weak, powerful, cruel, ignorant, finite, infinite, and mortal become immortal. This is the most baffling phase of Yoga and the least understood by modern philosophers.

To understand postoperative and postmeditative suggestions, we must explain the mechanism of concentration. In the meditative state, the subconscious mind is opened. All records of previous lives come into play. By the power of attention, all evil records are removed from the storehouse of the subconscious mind, and replaced with divine records. Evil life is removed and replaced with divine life. The result is that the entire personality is changed. In the state of meditation, the constant process of vivification and revivification is taking place. All lower desires are replaced by higher desires, ignorance by knowledge, unreality by reality, untruth by truth, and mortality by immortality. When meditation is over, one record is ready.

Now the postoperative and postmeditative record begins to play smoothly and constantly in our lives. It is the duty of the student to give this record freedom. In the meditative phase, the subconscious mind has recorded all commands, and after the meditation is over, postoperative and postmeditative suggestions begin to play in our lives. Many strange, incredible changes and happenings take place in our lives. The beginner will be spellbound by these transformations.

Usually people ask me how much time they should devote to meditation. My reply is: 24 hours per day and 365 days per year. They are perplexed by this answer. The classification is as follows:

When *nādam* is present, in meditation we check our evil habits and replace them by postmeditative suggestions. Process of postmeditative suggestions: "Oh, my subconscious mind: after you come to the conscious plane, I command you to make all sensory and motor organs strong and powerful. My conscious mind must have all extrasensory perceptions. I must not repeat the same mistakes again and again. My ears should not be ready to listen to evil sounds; my eyes should not see evil things; my tongue should not speak untruth; my hands should not do wrong work; my feet should not walk in a wrong direction, and all my sensory and motor organs must be free from all evil sensations and movements." In short, you must command your mind to virtuous performance and you have to give orders to check all evil movements of the body, senses, and mind.

The subconscious mind is a faithful servant. It follows every command, whether evil or divine. The order should come from your heart, not your tongue. The subconscious mind will not obey you if you command it verbally, and at the same time give your heart consciousness to do evil acts. Be sure that the subconscious mind receives the command from the heart, and not only from the tongue or other organs if they are not in agreement with the heart.

Therefore, in the meditative state, your heart should command your subconscious mind. After a few months' practice you will note that your mind is ready to follow your postmeditative orders, and thus your meditation is going on 24 hours per day, even while you are occupied in doing your daily work.

Do not place hindrances in the way of your subconscious mind while it is carrying out postmeditative suggestions. Sometimes you will feel conflicting forces of the subconscious and conscious minds. Give priority to all virtuous conscious and subconscious forces, and check all opposite forces. In this way you will be able to control all opposite forces and your mind will be free to carry out your orders. Do not request but command it.

Here we have to understand our daily life and the power

of our subconscious mind. Our daily life is filled with posthypnotic suggestions. Each and every moment we give suggestions for future work. For instance, when we awaken in the morning, we give suggestions to our subconscious mind for the entire day's work. When we study in school, we give suggestions to help us obtain a degree or diploma in the subject studied. When we make any program, we give suggestions for future work. Our lives are filled with hypnotic suggestions. If we are ready to remove the influence of hypnotism, we must give strong mental suggestions to dehypnotize our minds. Any habit, action, or performance is the result of previous suggestions to our subconscious mind; not only suggestions, but also the amount and intensity of previous suggestions are manifested in the degree and amount of our accomplishment. Therefore, in the meditative phase, give strong mental suggestions to your subconscious mind for the postmeditative phase.

If you do this, shortly you will feel that your subconscious mind is obeying you 24 hours per day, 365 days per year.

Your sleep will be according to your suggestions. You will have wonderful, splendid dreams. Postmeditative suggestions will brighten your life, and give you success, and consequently aid the world. Give affirmative suggestions, such as: "Each day I will be more relaxed; I will have more will power; each day I will be more successful; I will be happier; each day I will do more virtuous work; each day I will help others more and more; each day I will progress; each day I will conquer all my difficulties and see new visions in my meditation; each day I will be more successful in conquering my lust, lower desires, anger, and ignorance. In each meditation I will receive new life and new light. Each meditation will be progressive and will open a new field of vision. Each day I will improve my health and conquer my weakness, diseases, and sufferings."

These are a few affirmative postoperative and postmeditative suggestions. According to your situation, you can make innumerable suggestions to conquer your difficulties in time.

Lastly, your experience will be that you are able to dominate your subconscious mind, have it obey all your conscious commands. This is not a new thing for your subconscious mind. It obeys you every moment but you do not feel it.

Previously you gave wrong suggestions, which produced the negative results in your life, and now you think that your subconscious mind is against you. The subconscious mind is not against you, but your own previous negative suggestion is against your present situation. Our present life is the result of suggestions during our previous life, and our future life will be the result of present suggestions. If you want a good, successful future life and enlightenment, command your subconscious mind by enlightening suggestions.

This is the end of the fourteenth lesson. Read it, understand it, enlarge it, practice it, and enjoy the results of post-meditative suggestions.

15

ANESTHESIA PRODUCED BY YOGANIDRA

By means of concentration, anesthesia, one of the states of *yoganidra,* can be produced in any part of the body. This state can be produced locally or generally. The person who is in this state does not feel any pain.

Anesthesia is subjective and objective. When you produce it in yourself, it is subjective, and when in others, it is objective.

First, relax any particular part of your body, and when it is relaxed, magnetize it fully. Give strong suggestions that a particular part will feel no pain. Direct your will power firmly and you will note that that part is sensationless. You can produce anesthesia in any part of your body, or in any person. You must give strong *saṃyāmaḥ* (fixation, suggestion, and sensation) that any determined part of the body will feel no pain. You can select any sensitive part of the body, such as the tongue, ear, hand, foot, abdomen, etc. By consistent mental suggestions, that part becomes sensationless and you can now push a needle through it or operate upon it, and you will feel no sensation whatever. If a person is trained properly, there will be no need of injections or chloroform to produce local or general anesthesia if an operation is urgent. Any particular part of the body will be so sensationless that even a burning candle will not produce any pain reaction. In the beginning you may feel difficulty in doing this, but if you train yourself properly and practice regularly, you will be successful in anesthetizing any part or your entire body; it will be commonplace. When you observe the wonderful results of your practice, you will have great confidence in yourself and in your future progress, and future experiments will be easier for you.

Never make a show. Practice privately. Teach those who are sincere. By this method you will acquire power of tolerance for pain, pressure, touch, temperature, and they will not disturb your highest state of *samādhi*. Pain, pressure, touch, temperature, cold, etc., can disturb meditation and concentration, but after you have developed the technique to control them, they cannot disturb you.

> The mind comes under perfect control. It is free from all material desires and is absorbed in Supreme Consciousness. It is as seemingly motionless as an electric lamp and projects constant light. When, through the practice of Yoga, the mind ceases its restless movements and becomes still, the student realizes identity with the ocean of Supreme Consciousness. It satisfies him completely and he realizes that the happiness and peace obtained through Yoga is unique and without comparison. In his heart he realizes that the enjoyment obtained through Yoga is beyond the grasp of the senses. He stands firm in his realization, and because of it, he can never again wander away from the inmost truth of his being. He holds it as his treasurehouse, above all others. Even the deepest sorrow cannot disturb his presence of mind. It breaks all contact with aches and pains. You must practice it resolutely, without becoming discouraged. Renounce all material desires and practice it.—Gita, Chapter 6.

This is the end of the fifteenth lesson. Reread it, understand it, and practice it carefully to see the results of this chapter on your body.

Patiently, little by little, free yourself from all mental distractions with the aid of will power. Fix your mind on supreme consciousness, give strong suggestions, and feel that you have lost the consciousness of your body and you have identified yourself with supreme consciousness. If the restless and unquiet mind wanders, check it and fix it again on supreme consciousness. Within a few months' practice you will find yourself well established in the identity of the supreme and you will conquer all pains and sufferings of the body.

N O T E : There are certain drugs that produce local and general anesthesia, such as cocaine, novocaine, ether, chloroform, menthol, etc., but there is no spiritual evolution, no change in behavior; man is the same before and after anesthesia—while in and after Yoga anesthesia a sinner becomes a saint, a restless person becomes restful, and a man has the highest peace and happiness in his mind.

16

ṢATKARMAS: SIX METHODS TO REMOVE MENTAL AND PHYSICAL DISEASES

There are six techniques to remove mental and physical diseases, and when the body is free from diseases, it is enlightened by Self Consciousness:

1. *Dhauti*
2. *Basti*
3. *Neti*
4. *Trāṭakam*
5. *Naulikarma* or *Nauli*
6. *Kapala bhāti*

These six kinds of activities cleanse the body from all diseases, develop powerful senses for extrasensory perception, and enlighten the mind for Self Consciousness. These methods should be kept secret, should be practiced in a private place, and only under the guidance of an expert.

1. *Dhauti karm:* A strip of fine cloth about three inches wide and 15 feet long, moistened with warm water, should be swallowed slowly, and taken out again. It is swallowed progressively. Beginners should accomplish this process in 15 days. Each day one foot more of cloth should be swallowed progressively. For instance, the first day one foot, the second day two feet, etc., and the fifteenth day 15 feet. After swallowing the strip of cloth, a circular motion should be made, from left to right and from right to left, and then the cloth should be taken out slowly and gently. By this process the entire gastrointestinal tract (alimentary canal) is washed and all gastrointestinal diseases are

conquered. This is called *dhauti*—cleansing. The entire metabolism is improved by this process.

2. *Basti:* There are two types of *basti:*
   a. *Uttara basti.* To wash sex organs.
   b. *Adho basti.* To wash rectum.

   Pure water or milk is pumped into urinal bladder with a syringe. This process is repeated again and again. Saline or distilled water may be used. This is called *uttara basti.* In females, the entire vaginal path is irrigated by this method.

   Process: Take a piece of hose 6 inches in length, having a center opening of half an inch. The canal should pass through the entire length of the hose. Rub one end of the hose with oil or any other ointment and introduce it slowly into the rectum through anal canal. Sit in a tub that has previously been filled with water. The entire abdomen with anus should be contracted and the water should be drawn up and then expelled. This washing is called *adho basti.* An enema pot may be used for this purpose. Instead of water, milk and whey should be used with enema pot.

   Uttara basti removes all genital diseases, and *adho basti* removes all intestinal diseases; the senses are enlightened and digestion is increased.

3. *Neti:* A soft cord made of threads about six inches long should be passed slowly through the passage of the nose and taken out through the mouth. This is called *neti.* Force should be avoided. One nostril is always opened widely. Try it with relatively widened nostril. This cleans the entire head and, by reflex action, it stimulates the whole nervous system. It destroys the sinus diseases, neck diseases, and different headaches.

4. *Trāṭakam:* See Chapter 6.

5. *Nauli:* Place your hands on hips and bend your chest forward. Move abdominal muscles upward, downward, to the right, and to the left, alternately. After a few months' practice you will be able to do *nauli.* Move the abdomen forcefully. In this process the abdomen acts as a churning machine. This should

not be done in acute abdominal diseases nor in pregnancy. It removes all abdominal and chest diseases, stimulates metabolism, and gives perfect health.

6. *Kapala bhāti:* Inhale and exhale quickly and smoothly, like a pair of blacksmith bellows. This is called *kapala bhāti*. When you feel giddiness and dizziness, stop it and meditate. Do this more than once daily, but not more than five times per day in the beginning. This will remove all diseases from the head and central nervous system.

NOTE: *Śatkarma* should be performed only according to a teacher's instructions and with an expert on this subject.

This is the end of the sixteenth lesson. Read it, understand it, and practice it slowly and carefully.

*

17

THE SENSES AND EXTRASENSORY PERCEPTION

CLASSIFICATION OF SENSORY PERCEPTION

Sensation may conveniently be divided into:

1. Special sensory perception
2. General sensory perception
3. Extrasensory perception

The first is that which is appreciated by highly specialized nerve endings localized in certain parts of the body which are called sense organs, such as the nose, ear, eye, tongue, and skin. The second is not thus confined, and the third belongs to the highly developed consciousness.

General sensation is that felt by the body generally. It may be superficial, from the skin, and from the underlying structures of the body. If the nerves to the skin are cut or disintegrated by concentration, deep sensation remains. Superficial sensation consists of touch, pain, and temperature. Deep sensation is the appreciation of pressure that is distinct from touch or movement of the body and organs, or pain in the muscles and joints. The nerve fibers serving this sense run with the muscular nerves and accompany the blood vessels.

Extrasensory perception is the monopoly of concentration.

Various attempts have been made to classify sensation according to the mode of recovery of sensation in the section of the cutaneous nerves in the human body. All are agreed that crude sensation, such as produced by damage to the skin or extremes of temperature, is released first and is sufficient to produce generally protective movements. Later on, detailed localization, discrimination, and finer degrees of sensation return. Such division and subdivision of sensation are supported by researches in comparative anatomy and physiology, and it is directly perceived by our consciousness, which we obtain in the evolution of the nervous system through the process of concentration.

The nerve severely crushed recovers much more rapidly than one cut. An ordinary man has a highly developed mechanism, a general and special perception against a harmful environment. Later on, extrasensory perceptions and powers of discrimination are developed through the practice of Yoga. These sensations are intimately related to the acquisition of better motor control and vision, and with the expansion of the *śirobrahman* (cerebrum) or *sahasrāram,* an increasing understanding of all perceptions is developed. Be sure that each higher stage overlaps, reacts upon, and modifies the lower one. In short, each higher stage is the development of a lower one.

In discussing the general functions of the nervous system, you must remember that it is concerned with the collection of impulses resulting from stimuli in the individual, as well as the universal environment, and from the various parts of the body. A certain number of these impulses reach the field of consciousness and give rise to sensation. All sensations have limitations, and below and above that limitation they cannot grasp the impulses and, consequently, there will be no sensation beyond and below that limit. Hence, all sensations experienced normally depend on excitation by an appropriate stimulus of nerve-endings that are adapted to receive certain kinds of stimuli or to appreciate a special quality of the environment.

These nerve endings have, for the special stimulus for which they are adapted, a lower threshold than have the nerve fibers themselves, and make possible the setting up of a nerve impulse by a degree of stimulation that would not otherwise be effective. For instance, a degree of pressure that would not affect the ulnar nerve (the bone of the elbow) will cause a sensation of touch if applied to the nerve endings of that nerve in the little finger.

Nerve endings have been developed for the appreciation

of a large variety of stimuli, such as light, color, smell and pressure, etc.

Stimuli must not only have a special quality, but adequate strength. Too light a touch and too faint a sound will produce no effect on consciousness. That strength of stimulus which just suffices to evoke a sensation is called the liminal value of the stimulus, or its absolute threshold. Stimulus has a limit of duration also. This is well seen in relation to the eye. Movies appear continuous because they are changed very quickly, and if this does not occur, flicks are seen. Quickness of the hand deceives the eye. Similarly, the difference between two stimuli must not fall below a limit; otherwise the difference will not be appreciated. If two musical tones are of too nearly identical pitch, if two colors are of too nearly identical hues, the difference will be imperceptible. There is, therefore, a liminal value for a stimulus difference. This is known as the differential threshold of the stimulus.

Appreciable difference between two stimuli depends on the ratio of that difference to their magnitudes, and not on the absolute difference between their magnitudes. A rushing light will brighten a dark cellar, but its presence is unfelt in sunshine. So, too, if a room be lighted by a hundred candles and one more candle be brought in, the increased illumination produced by the extra candle would be just perceptible to the eye. But if a room were lighted by a thousand candles, no appreciable difference would result from the presence of an extra candle. Ten candles would have to be introduced in order to effect a just noticeable difference. In each case a difference of one hundredth of the original strength of stimulus is necessary to cause a just appreciable difference in the sensation. For light, the fraction is about one hundredth, as stated above; for sound it is about one third; for cutaneous pressure it varies between one thirtieth and one tenth; for weight, between one seventieth and one fortieth in various parts of the body.

Appreciable time is required for the development of sensation. Part of this time is spent at the end organs on which the stimulus acts, part in conveying the impulse along the sensory nerve to the brain, and part within the brain itself. This latent period varies in length according to the sensation, e.g., it is longer for sight than for sound and longer for pain than for touch.

The sensation outlasts its stimulus. Such after-sensations are particularly noticeable in the case of sight. If we look at an object intently, we can continue to see it for a time after we close our eyes.

The Impulse. The nerve impulse is identical in nature in all nerves. The nerve impulse set up in the optic nerve by light is the same as that set up in the auditory nerve by sound. The difference in sensation is recognized by the individual through "analyzers" present in the central nervous system. The impulses reaching certain analyzers, such as those of sight, are interpreted as light however the impulse is set up. Every sense organ, however excited, gives rise to its own specific sensation. However the retina or optic nerve is stimulated, light is appreciated. Mechanical, chemical, or electrical stimulation of the Chorda Tympane causes a sensation of taste.

The skin plays a principal part in all sensation. The whole body is the manifestation of ectoderm, mesoderm, and endoderm. The skin has the following functions:

1. Protection.
2. Sensation.
3. Heat regulation.
4. Respiration.
5. Absorption of nutrient substance.
6. Blood depot.
7. Secretion of sweat (hot and cold secretions).
8. Sebum or oil substance.
9. Storehouse for hair.
10. Storehouse for pigmentation.
11. Storehouse of beauty, etc.

By the process of concentration, all perceptions are increased. Limitation is broken. The student of Yoga can go below or above the limitation. Physiological limitations are for an ordinary man. He who concentrates according to Yoga has clairvoyance and clairaudience. His general sensations, special sensations, and extrasensory perceptions are unique.

The beginner must now be in a position to perceive a

clearer, more comprehensive picture of the functions of the central nervous system (*suśumna*) as a whole. Throughout the animal kingdom it exists for the purpose of regulating the internal mechanism of the body and for adapting the activities of the body as a whole to its environment. As we ascend the zoological scale, the animals become increasingly capable of adapting themselves to different kinds of environment; this is very largely due to their greater capability of locomotion, which in a sense is considered the index of evolution. By examining the entire animal kingdom you will come to the conclusion that the nervous system is developed largely according to locomotory requirements.

A simple animal such as a jellyfish, which does not move much from place to place, has a nervous system capable only of protecting itself. It has a nerve net in which the essential elements of a simple reflex are found: that is, sensory fibers, central cells, and motor fibers.

Slightly higher animals, e.g., worms, which move but slightly more, have a central chain of ganglia; each ganglion looks after a segment, but there is co-operation among the ganglia for the protection of the whole. This is the basal function of the spinal cord and brainstem of mammals.

As the animals become still more mobile, they require some arrangement for a greater supply of *prāṇa vāyu* (air) and food; then the medulla and pons are developed, in which are situated the centers to control respiration and circulation. The faculty of digestion is increased by the vagal activity (tenth cranial nerve) controlling swallowing, secretions, and alimentary movements. A vomiting center is developed for protection against noxious substances swallowed through the alimentary canal.

With still greater mobility conferred by the acquisition of the legs are developed the postural reflexes controlled from the upper part of the medulla to the mid-brain, and greater co-ordination is provided by the development of the *śirobalam* (cerebellum) in close association.

In still higher animals, there are in the hypothalamus centers that confer adaptation to variations of temperature, and all the advantages of rapid chemical and mechanical actions that the warm-blooded animals possess. This region is included in the *ājñā cakram* and it is regarded as the center of the primitive system that has as its function the preservation of the individual and his species. By this region, with the association of *somamaṇḍalam* (pituitary gland), reproduction and growth are controlled. The more violent reactions to environment are located here.

The *śirobrahman* (cerebrum) is developed in the highest animals, and it relates past to present experience and permits of calculated adaptation to still more complicated environments. By means of modern mechanical transportation and communication, still greater mobility of body and thought is arranged by it.

As regards slower but constant reactions, the ductless glands furnish still further adaptations: the pituitary for growth and reproduction, the thyroid for metabolic control, adrenal for all minute activities, and other endocrine glands are developed to provide special actions, movements, adaptations, and sensations.

As we ascend we find that the influence of the individual on the environment becomes increasingly greater. At one end of the scale there is the creature that dies when there is any appreciable environmental change, and at the other end of the scale there is man who, while capable of greater adaptation than the lower animals, is at the same time beyond them in being the creator and master of a large section of his environment.

Methods. The aim of Yoga is to examine all sensations and to increase all perceptions up to the level of perfection. For this reason you must have a working knowledge of the anatomy and physiology of all the senses, sensory and motor pathways, sensory organs, sensory centers, and psychic centers.

The principal aim of concentration is to awaken *kuṇḍalinī* (nervous system) sleeping within the limit of the threshold. All hormonal secretions are preserved from misuse and are transformed for the development of the nervous system. Through the power of *saṃyamaḥ* (fixation, suggestion, and sensation), the limiting threshold is uplifted and man begins to feel the entire phenomenon of supreme nature.

Place your body in a comfortable posture. Relax the entire body. Practice *pratyāhāra* (withdrawal of energy). Withdraw energy and consciousness from every organ and limb and feel the change in sensations. For practice, take first one part of the body, then another. Turn your whole body into *yoganidra.* Magnetize it fully. Feel electromagnetic waves around and within you. If you do not feel this, relax your body again completely. Practice holding your breath and with great attention feel general, special, and extrasensory perceptions. The body becomes very sensitive, the mind becomes more penetrative and the senses become more acute.

Extrasensory perception does not depend on senses. It is the monopoly of consciousness. When supreme consciousness is manifested, you have exact knowledge of yourself and the universe around you. No doubt sometimes this perception is opened to an ordinary man and he begins to know much that has previously been concealed, but this is momentary and beyond his control. Everyone may have this type of experience in his lifetime, but the extrasensory perceptions obtained through Yoga are permanent and under control and they lead to perfection.

For special extrasensory perception meditate on *nādam;* practice *trāṭakam;* practice the nasal gaze.

Through practice, the whole nervous system is awakened and the body becomes a small moving universe. In this body you have everything: the world, suns, moons, stars you see outside you can also see within yourself by the power of *samādhi.* Your body will be the true receiver and transmitter to send motor power and to receive sensations. You will have a moving broadcasting station in your central nervous system.

This is the end of the seventeenth lesson. Read it, understand it. Enlarge it by your commentary and concentrate your mental powers, and perceive the wonderful drama of *kuṇḍalinī śakti* (coiled potential power), when it is awakened from the sleeping state.

18

HOW TO OPEN THE THIRD EYE

Introduction. The third eye is located in the center of the forehead. The third eye and the exact location of the third eye—that is to say, the forehead, the point starting from between the eyebrows and reaching up to the center of the forehead—is a symbolic description in Yoga. It is triangular in form, its base between the eyebrows and vertex in the center of the forehead. The third eye is representative of eternal knowledge, and the place is representative of *ājñā cakram.* The thalamus with all its endocrine glands and nerve connections, regarded as the seat of individual consciousness and with duct connection to the cerebral cortex (*sahasrāram*)—that is to say, the cerebral cortex—exercises its power all over the body through this center. This place is selected for the purpose of practice. In addition, this is not only the anatomical location but also a psychic *cakram,* which includes all those structures of the central nervous system responsible for individual personality, and existence, and knowledge. In the ordinary state, this center is working partially. Through learning and modern philosophy it works moderately, but through the practice of Yoga it operates fully and perfectly. The awakening of this *cakram* is technically termed the opening of the third eye. It is not an eye in that sense in which we have our muscular eyes. It is called an eye because through it we see exactly our own true form and the universe around us. It is third in number because we already have two eyes to see the physical world.

General Description. During my tour throughout the

world, many people came to ask me this question, and because I am also an M.D., they are particularly interested in learning something from me. The question is: "Is it possible to open the third eye by an operation?" Not only this, but in India many people came to my consultation office who were very curious about the third eye and were ready for and desirous of an operation, if it were possible. They brought various collections of clippings from all over the world, and from many books written by a variety of authors regarding this subject. My answer is very clear and simple: "Yes." With this positive answer people became very hopeful, happy, and ready for an operation. But when I explained the real meaning of operation, its process and cost, up to date they have seldom returned.

No doubt the third eye is opened by operation, but this operation can never be performed in hospitals. For this operation you need a living area full of spiritual atmosphere. As in the operating room, we need a surgeon, assistant surgeons, anesthetist, and other helpers. In this operation our surgeon is *anāhat nādam*, or eternal mind. The operating table is an easy posture; general anesthesia is produced by the power of *saṃyamaḥ* (fixation, suggestion, and sensation). All the sensory and motor organs are assistants here. All other environmental situations are helpers here. This is the most difficult operation in the world. When, through the power of *saṃyamaḥ*, the body is magnetized and completely anesthetized by *pratyāhāra* (withdrawal of energy and consciousness), one becomes ready for this operation. If anesthesia is superficial, the operation cannot be done. Therefore, one should go into the deepest state of *samādhi*. This is the deepest anesthesia. In this state the subconscious mind opens all its previous records and the power of attention removes all evil impressions recorded in the subconscious mind. Thus, when ignorance is removed, intuition begins to work without obstruction. Intuition naturally has the power of penetration, but it is prevented from exercising its power by our ignorance.

Method or Technique.

1. Place your body in a comfortable posture so that if deep sleep comes, your body will not fall from that

posture. Otherwise, you may hurt yourself and disturb your process.

2. Remove all anxieties and weakness from your mind.
3. Think that behind this body is operating an eternal energy, which has created innumerable stars, moons, and planets, and it is your own nature.
4. Now this eternal energy is shining around us. Its power is radiating throughout the world. Think a few minutes of it.
5. Slowly close your eyes and fix your attention over the whole body. Think strongly that you are going to anesthetize your whole body. Use *saṃyamaḥ* and the power of *pratyāhāra.* Relax your whole body, withdraw energy from every organ, and fix it on the place of the third eye. Listen constantly to *nādam.* Fix your will power on the center of the forehead.
6. Remain in this state until you feel that you have no body. You will forget every part of your body and feel identity with supreme consciousness. In this state you will receive the highest intuition and penetrating will power.
7. When you are in this state, *nādam* will remove ignorance forever and you will see the dawn of eternal knowledge in the firmament of the mind. This is called the third eye, and this process is the operation to open that eye.

NOTE: If in your process your experimentation is disturbed, never mind, but repeat this process again in the same way. After a few months' practice you will feel that you are on the right path to open your third eye. For a complete operation you will take a long time. It is most difficult but not impossible. The human body is the only body authorized to open this eye. By your perseverance and patience, you will be successful in the long run. To accomplish your practice quickly, you must have a working knowledge of anatomy, physiology, and Yoga psychology.

This is the end of the eighteenth lesson. Here is the brief method of opening your third eye. Read it, understand it. If you do not understand, consult your teacher or an expert on this subject. When you fully understand the method, be your own surgeon to open your third eye.

19

AWAKEN YOUR KUNDALINĪ

Before going into the study of the different direct methods of inducing the state of *samādhi,* it is now important that you should understand how to awaken your *kuṇḍalinī śakti.*

Introduction. Every soul is potentially divine and eternal. It is in potential form; hence it is called, figuratively, in sleeping state. When it awakens, it manifests chain reactions and actions; therefore it is called *kuṇḍalinī śakti* (coiled energy). Individual *kuṇḍalinī śakti* (coiled energy) is the manifestation of universal *kuṇḍalinī śakti;* therefore, it is eternal and immortal. In the ordinary states it is operating partially. In educated and trained persons it operates moderately. In the state of *samādhi* it operates fully and perfectly.

General Description. Before going into the study of awakening your *kuṇḍalinī śakti* (potential Self), it is important that you understand the *kuṇḍalinī* path and its relation with *suśumna, suśumna śirśakam, suśumnakand, śirobalab,* and *śirobrahman.*

The *kuṇḍalinī* path is the mechanism that deals with the correlation and integration of various bodily processes, the reaction and adjustments of the organism to its environment and with the conscious, superconscious, and subconscious life. It may be regarded as the nervous system as a whole. From a practical point of view, it is classified into two parts: *suśumna* (central nervous system) and *parisariya naḍi manḍalam* (peripheral nervous system). The central nervous system or *suśumna* consists of the *śirobrahman*

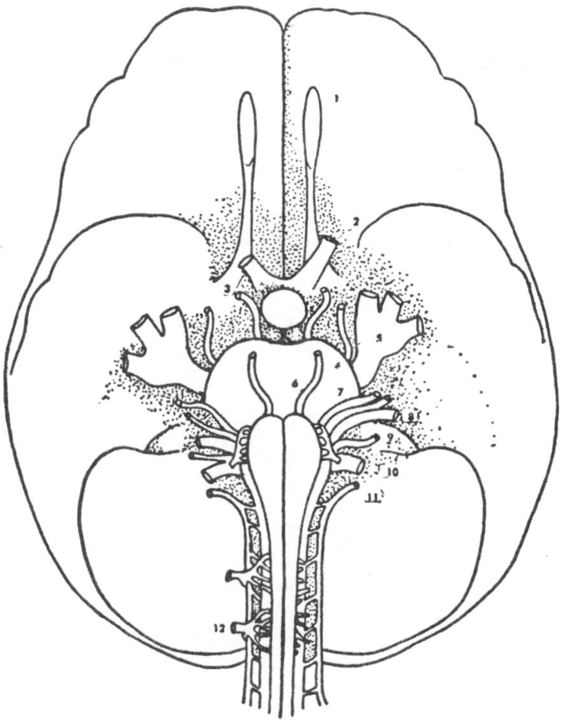

Courtesy, The CIBA Collection of Medical Illustrations, Volume I

IV

CRANIAL NERVES

1. Olfactory
2. Optic
3. Oculomotor
   (All eye muscles except those below, also iris sphincter, ciliary)
4. Trochlear
   (Superior oblique)
5. Trigeminal
   (Sensory to face, sinuses, teeth, etc., masticator nerve to muscles of mastication)
6. Abducens
   (External rectus)
7. Facial
   (Muscles of face)
   (Glossopalatine, n. intermedius. Motor to submaxillary and sublingual gl. Sensory—anterior part of tongue and soft palate)
8. Acoustic
   auditory
   vestibular
9. Glossopharyngeal
   (Sensory—posterior part of tongue, tonsil, pharynx
   Motor—pharyngeal musculature)
10. Vagus
   (Motor—heart, lungs, bronchi, g.i. tract
   Sensory—heart, lungs, bronchi, trachea, larynx, pharynx, g.i. tract, external ear)
11. Accessory
   Sternomastoid
   Trapezius
12. Hypoglossal
   Tongue muscles

(cerebrum) contained within the cranium, the *śirobalam* (cerebellum), the *suśumna śirśakam* (medulla oblongata), and the *suśumna kandam* (spinal cord lodged in the vertebral canal). In all parts *suśumna* is continuous.

The *parisariya nadi maṇḍalam* (peripheral nervous system) consists of a series of nerves by which the *suśumna* (central nervous system) is connected with the various tissues of the body. It is classified into three groups:

1. Cranial.
2. Spinal.
3. Autonomic nervous system.

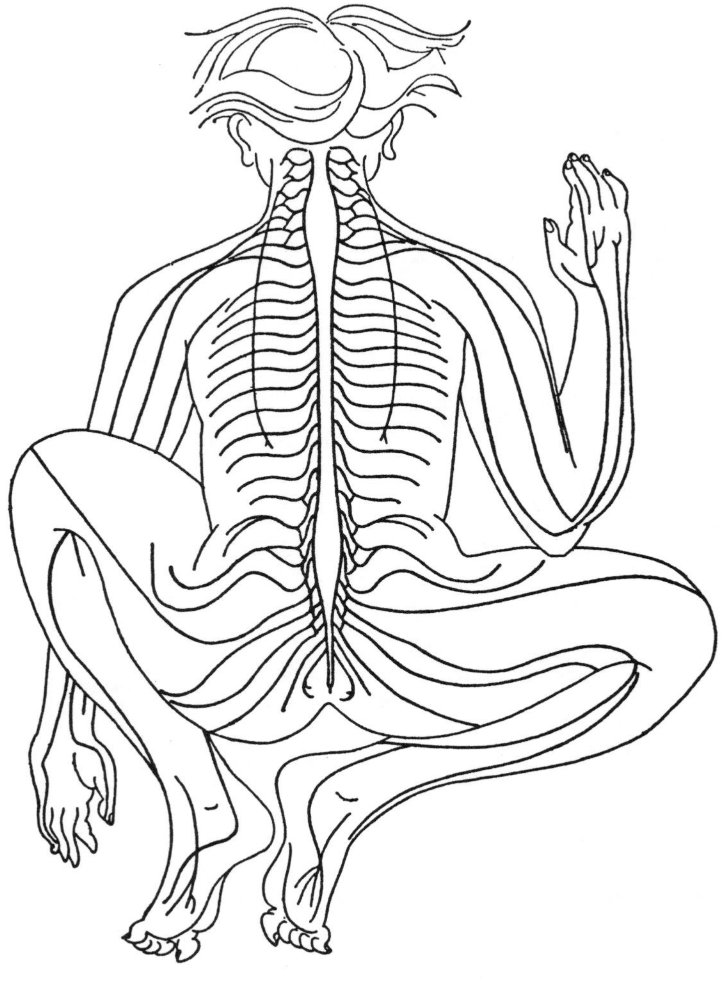

V

CENTRAL AND PERIPHERAL NERVOUS SYSTEM

This line drawing is intended to show the essential ramifications of the nervous system. A diagram on this scale can not indicate the many numerous and fine nerves radiating from the spinal cord. The nervous system as a whole is the Kuṇḍalinī Path.

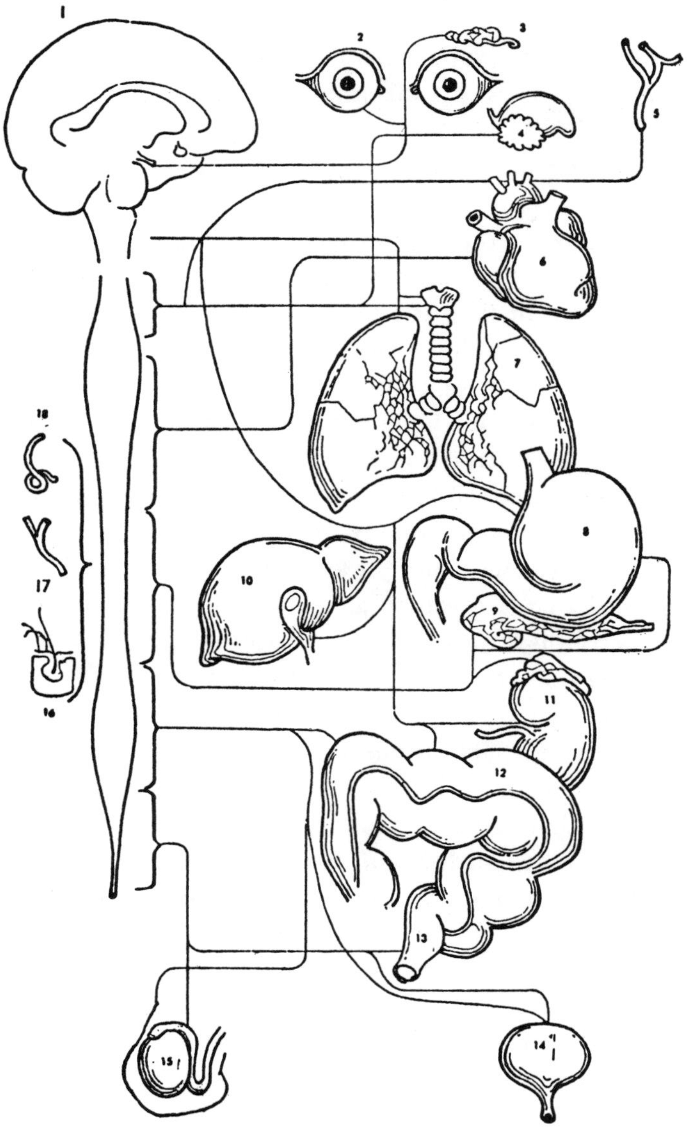

VI

THE AUTONOMIC NERVOUS SYSTEM AND ITS RELATION TO THE CENTRAL NERVOUS SYSTEM

The central nervous system as a whole is called SUŚUMNA and the autonomic nervous system is called IDA (parasympathetic nervous system) and PINGALA (sympathetic nervous system).

1. Central nervous system, or SUŚUMNA
2. Eyes
3. Lachrymal glands
4. Salivary glands
5. Intra-cranial vessels
6. Heart
7. Larynx, trachea, bronchi and lungs
8. Stomach
9. Pancreas
10. Liver and gall bladder
11. Adrenals and kidneys
12. Intestines
13. Colon
14. Bladder
15. Gonads
16. Hair follicle
17. Peripheral vessel
18. Sweat gland

The entire nervous system is derived from ectodermal cells. The process of awakening is as follows:

1. Place your body in a comfortable posture.
2. Relax yourself up to the third state.
3. Think of the whole nervous system: that you are able to magnetize your entire body through the *kuṇḍalinī* path (nervous system).
4. Use the whole hormonal power to strengthen your *kuṇḍalinī* system.
5. Feel that your body is full of pulsation and electromagnetic attraction.
6. Forget the feeling of the body and identify yourself with *Brahman* (supreme consciousness).
7. Feel that life and light are flowing from you.
8. Feel that a great ocean of consciousness and magnetism is flowing in you and around you.
9. Feel that you are the supreme Self.
10. Feel that you are the power of the entire universe.
11. Perceive that innumerable stars, suns, and planets are in you.
12. Feel that you are liberated and exalted.
13. Feel that you have no body, no material mind, no lust, no anger, no hatred, and no enmity toward anybody.
14. Feel that the entire universe is in you and you are in the entire universe.
15. Listen attentively to the *anāhata nādam* sound everywhere.

After practicing a long time, you will feel that you are on the right way, and after great effort, your *kuṇḍalinī śakti* will awaken and lead your consciousness from the individual field to universal consciousness. You will feel the highest, inexpressible enjoyment in yourself. The whole universe will be your home. All old relations will be changed; you will have a feeling of being at home, and as if one soul were in everything. Only the mind can experience it, but the tongue and pen cannot describe it.

This is the end of the nineteenth lesson. Read it. Consult an anatomical and physiological chart to understand it. Practice it and verify it.

20

HEAL YOURSELF BY YOUR OWN HORMONES AND TRANQUILIZERS

In the field of education this is the age of science, but in the field of human life this is the age of tranquilizers and hormones. The real principle of treatment is too little known to the world. Symptomatic treatment is going on. Very few pay any attention to removing the cause of the disease. Symptoms are the partial manifestation of the disease and not the disease itself. Doctors are busy in treating the disease, but they must learn to treat the patient as a whole, rather than the disease. New research is going on daily in the medical field, but the study of the patient lags far behind. For instance, if a patient has a pain in his body or has the condition of sleeplessness, analgesic and hypnotic drugs are given, respectively, to alleviate the symptoms and the real cause of the disease is most frequently neglected. Consequently, amputation of limbs and removal of organs are carried out for the diseased part, and the patient with his sleeplessness becomes a potential life member of some mental institution. This is the great drawback in modern treatment. The more treatment, the more serious the condition of the patient becomes.

Daily new hormones are arriving on the market, which are supposed to have a magical influence on disease, but no one is ready to treat himself by means of his own hormones. If hormones of dead animals can exert tremendous influence and temporarily cure a patient, then why cannot your own hormones cure your physical and mental disease permanently? Dead glands are kept in refrigeration and chemical hormones are extracted from these frozen glands. But if you use human glands, your own glands, while they are in a living state, the result will be far more constructive. But you do not know how to use your own hormones in the living state of the body. The practice of Yoga teaches you how to use your own hormones and your own endocrine glands while they are in the living state in your body.

Many people are uninformed or misinformed on the subject of healing, and some professional healers aid their peculiar confusion. When you depend only on others for your healing, you may be temporarily healed to some extent, but your mind is degenerating progressively on the subconscious level. When the disease returns, this type of healing process is less effective and the patient is forced to seek more extreme forms of treatment. New devices are invented daily to treat the symptoms of disease, but the real causes of many diseases are not known sufficiently, if at all; often they are rooted in the personality of the patient. A knowledge of Yoga psychology, even in the early stages, teaches you how to co-operate with your own medical doctor, who has objective knowledge of anatomy, the nervous system, the endocrine system, etc. The medical doctor is a student and a dedicated person; he is very necessary and those who belittle his efforts and his interest in helping them are truly foolish. Your development psychologically can help him to use his knowledge more productively in your own behalf; the study of Yoga is in no way antithetical to the purposes of the professional medical doctor.

Yoga psychology teaches you how to heal yourself by your own hormones, how to tranquilize your mind by your own power of thought, how to extract your own hormones from your glands, how to prepare them to heal your mental and physical diseases, and how to develop your body, senses and the mind by them. It is difficult, but if we pay serious attention to the processes taught by Yoga psychology, at some future date we can obtain perfection from it.

According to Yoga psychology, thought is the manifestation of universal energy and, as an energy, it has two functions: construction and destruction, according to the use made of it. If we use it for higher thinking, we construct our body, senses, and mind, and if we use it for lower thinking, we destroy them.

By higher thinking the endocrine secretions that are constantly passing in the blood are utilized in the formation of *ojas śakti*. The essence of hormonal energy is called *ojas*. Your nervous system operates with the energy of *ojas*. There are two *ojas: para ojas,* which supplies the heart—when it is gone, life ends; and *apara ojas,* which circulates constantly through the blood vessels to nourish the entire body, to heal mental and physical diseases. When it is deficient, mental and physical diseases are manifest.

By constant thought energy, both *ojas* are utilized. They are misused if there is wrong thinking, the results of which are first presented in the psychological field, then in the physiological; and lastly in the form of mental and physical diseases in the pathological field, with the manifestation of innumerable symptoms.

Mental and physical natures are the result of what we have thought. Thought is the leader of our personality, behavior, and existence. Hatred will never cease in those who entertain thoughts of revenge. As the wind uproots a tree of little strength, so indeed do thoughts of lust, anger, and material desire overthrow those who harbor them in their minds, and he who yearns only for pleasures has no control over the senses, is immoderate in eating, indolent, and of low vitality. As the wind cannot blow down a rocky mountain, so *mārā* (lust) cannot overthrow those who live unmindful of pleasures, have control of their senses, are moderate in eating, are busy in the investigation of intuition, and are of high vitality.

As rain does not break through a well-constructed house, so passion does not make its way into a reflective mind. Thoughtlessness is the abode of death and suffering, and thoughtfulness is the cure and the abode of eternal life. Those who are vigilant do not die, but the thoughtless are already dead. Not a mother, nor a father, nor any other relation can do as much for us as a well-directed mind, which will do us the greatest service.

A man who frees himself from impure thoughts attains salvation. The total elimination of impure thoughts is possible only as a result of much *tapasya* (austerity). There is only one way to achieve it. Whenever an impure thought comes to the mind, it should immediately be confronted with a pure one. This, again, is possible only by the grace of *anāhata nādam* (*śabda brahman*). That grace is obtained by concentration and meditation on it. There will be no progress if OM is repeated verbally, while the mind is full of evil thoughts. OM should be repeated with such concentrated effort that what has remained on the lips so far will come, in the course of time, to occupy the first place in the mind. Again, however, much as the mind might try, it should not be given control over a single sense organ. A man who allows his senses to drift wherever the mind chooses to drag them must meet with destruction in the end. But as long as one keeps the sense organs even forcibly under self-control, one can hope some day to gain mastery over destructive thoughts. Even a well-controlled master of mind must follow these laws. The rise of impure thoughts should not be the cause of depression; on the contrary, it should inspire greater zeal in us. A wrongly directed mind will do us greater harm than an external enemy. Alas, this body will live on earth, despised, bereft of consciousness, a useless life, a heap of garbage.

Before post-mortem, do your own ante-mortem to check your mind. Those who control their thoughts, which travel far, incorporeal, seated in the mind and heart, will be able to free themselves from the fetters of death and diseases. True law and wisdom can not remain in an unsteady mind; and fear, anxiety, physical and mental diseases as cruel as death cannot attack a well-trained mind. If a person is reflective, if he rouses himself, if he is ever mindful, if his deeds are pure, if he acts with consideration, if he is self-restrained and lives according to the law, his glory will increase. The wise man, by rousing himself, by vigilance, by restraint, by control, makes for himself an island which the mighty ocean waves cannot overwhelm. By vigilance of thoughts, Indra rose to the lordship of the gods. The wise in all periods praise vigilance of thought, and thoughtlessness is always deprecated as death.

Process of Healing.

1. Place your body in a comfortable posture.
2. Relax your body.
3. Send strong *saṃyamaḥ* to remove unfavorable mental and physical conditions from your body and mind.
4. Think that they are going out of your body and mind.

5. Think that now your body and mind are free from all desire.
6. Now forget about the entire body and identify yourself with supreme consciousness. After a few days' practice you will feel that you have no feeling of your body, and instead of your body, you have a small electromagnetic station full of pulsation.
7. Remain in this state and think that all mental and physical diseases are healed. Feel it and you will see practically that they are healed.
8. Repeat this process in sunlight and feel that light and life from the sun are coming to nourish constantly all planets, as well as yourself.
9. Feel reaction of sunlight through your body.
10. Now feel that the body is hot: the entire solar system is filled with light and life.
11. Feel that you are the sun and giving light and life to every planet.
12. Remain in this state for a few minutes and you will note that your body is covered with sweat and all diseases are healed through radiation of sun rays.
13. Repeat this formula in the water when you have an opportunity to swim or bathe.
14. Repeat the same process when you take a shower or bath.
15. Imagine many situations according to your approach and repeat this process.

This is the end of the twentieth lesson. Read it. Consult an anatomical and physiological chart to familiarize yourself with the positions and functions of the endocrine glands, nervous system, and other organs. Study and practice. Preserve your hormonal secretions. Develop your *ojas* and heal yourself by yourself. You will be the best doctor to diagnose your mental and physical conditions and to treat them fully.

Examine your mind and thoughts constantly and lead them from darkness to light, from suffering to life, from death to mortality, from unreality to reality, and be happy. Eventually you will be your own doctor.

21 THE HEART AND CONSCIOUSNESS

Introduction.

1. The physical heart and physical consciousness are related.
2. In the same way, the spiritual heart and spiritual consciousness are related.

In physiological considerations of sensations and voluntary movements, it is extremely important to understand the real nature of consciousness, but physiologists are far from understanding its exact nature. Academically, physical consciousness belongs to biology and psychology, but it is becoming abundantly clear that there is no hard and fast line between the subjects of physiology, biology, and psychology.

The entire education, training, and behavior depend on consciousness. Biological or physical consciousness is defined as an awareness of the existence of one's self and of the external world, and the evidence is very complete that in man it is dependent on the occurrence of a given amount of oxidation taking place in the cerebrum. Without such chemical changes, we know that nerve cells cease to function and die. Life and consciousness are by-products of the heart. If the heart stops, life and consciousness cease to function and a being is pronounced dead.

Consciousness is a correlate of the activity of the cerebral nerve cells, and we are aware of certain streams of impulses that pass through the cerebrum, provided they are of sufficient magnitude, whether they occur during the waking or sleeping states. If they occur while we are asleep, a dream results and then we are not in the waking state.

The state of consciousness varies throughout the animal kingdom but in man alone has reached a stage of evolution that makes it possible for him to form mental concepts, of which the psychological concept is the most important.

But the story of consciousness is not over. Biological heart and consciousness are physical in nature and they depend on the metaphysical heart and consciousness. In reality, consciousness is not created but manifested, and this manifestation depends on the evolution of the nervous system. Consciousness is highly developed through the human nervous system but, according to changes in the nervous system and blood, it enters into such different states as waking, dreaming, and sound sleep.

When, through the practice of concentration, the nervous system is fully developed, consciousness is manifested in its full form, and one feels its eternal existence, eternal bliss. The cerebrum is not necessary for this consciousness. Biological consciousness depends upon the following factors:

1. The physical integrity of the brain.
2. The oxygen supply to the brain.
3. The blood supply to the brain.
4. The purity of the body and the senses.

If the above are disturbed, consciousness is reduced to different levels. Sleep, fatigue, and toxic conditions create changes in consciousness. But here you do not need to be concerned about the physical heart and consciousness. Your principal aim is to reach the spiritual heart and spiritual consciousness by means of the physical heart and physical consciousness.

Technique.

1. Adopt an easy posture.
2. Relax your entire body.
3. Feel your heart pumping in the chest.
4. Hold your breath.

5. In a moment you will feel that heart rate and vigor of beat are increased.
6. With every heartbeat, the heart is sending energy to every part of the body. Feel it.
7. With increased heart rate and beat, energy is changed into electromagnetic pulsation and the entire body is filled with it. Feel it.
8. The entire body is now magnetized, and the spiritual heart and spiritual consciousness are fully manifested in you. Feel them.
9. The whole body becomes the heart of the universe, and you feel that the entire body is pulsating as a single heart.
10. Gradually you forget the feelings of the physical body and you identify yourself completely with supreme consciousness.
11. Now you know that your consciousness is never a product of the body, but it is manifested in the body.
12. Feel that your body is one point of manifestation of consciousness, but really you are everywhere.
13. Feel that this body is not the center of your body; you can work through any body. After long practice you will feel that you can work through any body.
14. Feel that you are that consciousness, and you will be free.
15. Feel that it is eternal, and immortal, and you will have eternal knowledge, peace, bliss, and happiness.

This is the end of the twenty-first lesson. Read it. Consult an anatomical and physiological chart to understand the heart, blood vessels, and nervous system in order to increase your understanding for concentration. Practice daily on the spiritual heart and consciousness by means of physical heart and consciousness. After a few months' practice you will sense more of the healthy physical changes in yourself.

22

HOW TO CONTROL VITARKAS

Those activities of the mind which are wrong and destructive to our personality, senses, body, and mind are called *vitarkas.* Logically, philosophically, ethically, morally, socially, and legally we understand these wrong mental waves and recognize that they are disastrous to our existence; still, owing to their powerful hypnotic influence and force, we feel compelled to act according to them. This is called our own behavior against our real existence and personality. These cruel mental waves are called *vitarkas* (*vi,* against; *tarka,* reason, consciousness, logic, standard, philosophy, rationale) because they are against our reason, standard, logic, philosophy, and life.

From a practical point of view, they are summarized in ten groups, as follows:

1. Injury to others.
2. Untruthfulness, prejudice.
3. Stealing.
4. Incontinence.
5. Hoarding of money for selfish satisfaction.
6. Impurity of body, mind, and senses.
7. Discontentment.
8. Selfishness.
9. Indolence and stoppage of study.
10. No desire to work according to wisdom and intuition.

These ten groups are given here; you may enlarge them as much as you wish.

To control these *vitarkas,* you have two divine forces within you: *yama* and *niyama. Yama* is called a serious intention to control them. Many of our students and friends attend the Yoga lectures and classes to acquire a knowledge of Yoga psychology as a hobby or to satisfy their curiosity. They have no serious intention of becoming real Yogis, but they find that they can become the center of attraction at social affairs and among their friends by demonstrating their supernatural powers. Many modern so-called Yogis help them through advertisements, correspondence, and newspapers. Many students and Yogi enthusiasts have reported astonishing success among their friends. Many Western cities and provinces are congested with these miracles. But how many of these people seriously wish to control beneficially their minds and mental waves? This will be examined.

Yama means a serious intention to control the mind. Generally, everyone wants, superficially, to control the mind and to have some unusual powers, if possible, but their internal part of the mind gives constant concession to continue *vitarkas.* When the mind decides, internally, to control these waves, it is called *yama. Yama* means control, and becomes successful by following these five steps:

1. *Ahiṃsā:* Noninjury to others by body, speech, and mind.
2. *Satyam:* Promise to follow truth and to renounce untruth from one's life.
3. *Asteyam:* Nonstealing.
4. Continence: Control of hormonal powers to develop the body, senses, and mind through the development of *ojas.*
5. *Aparigraha:* No hoarding of money; to work as a manager of our own property. Ten per cent of our earnings belongs to others. If we donate 10 per cent of our property, it is good, but we still do not donate anything, because it belongs to others. When we donate more than 10 per cent, then we really serve the world. This is called *aparigraha.* If this were practiced properly, there would be no necessity to fear communism. A student of Yoga must decide that he will follow the ways of Yoga.

These five *yamas* enable the student to control the first five *vitarkas*. Even if we have serious intentions to control our minds, it does not help us if these are not in our daily practice. We must practice them seriously.

The following five *niyamas* will help your practice:

1. Purity of body, senses, and heart.
2. Contentment.
3. *Tapasya* (austerity).
4. *Śvādhyāya* (study of Yoga psychology and philosophy).
5. Transformation of the body into a worthy medium; self-surrender to wisdom, intuition, and consciousness.

Niyama means observances; to make successful one's intentions, or *yamas*. These five *niyamas* enable the student to control the last five *vitarkas*.

For each *vitarka* you have, you can create its opposite, and make your life successful.

There are five other methods to control mental waves:

1. An analysis of every problem and the search for its proper solution (this does not always work in the case of habits).
2. Neutrality. Observe your mental activities as a witness, not an agent; do not work as their agent, and control all waves.
3. Keep your life occupied.
4. *Bhāvasamādhi*. To forget the body and material mind, and to identify with supreme consciousness.
5. *Brahmi-sthiti*. "I am *Brahman*. The whole universe is *Brahman*. *Vitarkas* have no meaning for me."

You will select the way which is most suitable to you.

This is the end of the twenty-second lesson. Read it; understand it. Enlarge it by your commentary; search other methods. Observe them and make your life successful. Without the practice of *yama* and *niyama*, perfection is impossible. Practice them to control your *vitarkas*.

23

THE FIVE GREAT SUGGESTIONS

These are the five great Vedic suggestions to lead the mind from the world of name and form to perfection:

1. *Tattvamasi* (Thou art that).
2. *Aham Brahmāsmi* (I am Brahman).
3. *Ayamātmā Brahman* (This Self is Brahman).
4. *Prajñānam Brahman* (Consciousness is Brahman).
5. *Satcidānandam Brahman* (Eternal existence, eternal consciousness, eternal peace is Brahman).

1. *Tattvamasi.* The body is composed of two substances: nature and consciousness, or matter and mind. The natural elements of the body are the same as those of the universe; and the consciousness of the body is the same as that of the universe. Therefore, "thou art that" means thy consciousness is not individual but universal, and because universal consciousness and nature are eternal thy consciousness and natural elements are eternal. The main emphasis is on consciousness because it is the leader of the natural elements. When you go into deeper concentration you face dualism. That is to say, in the state of deep concentration you feel identity with supreme consciousness, which indicates thou art that, but when you come out of that state you have still individual consciousness, which indicates thou art this. What is the ultimate reality of the two? In this doubt "thou art that" indicates meditative experience as the ultimate and eternal truth because every high experience condemns the lower experience to the point of unreality.

2. *Aham Brahmāsmi.* (Here the term "I" is not used in a personal sense; it is impersonal and universal I.) In this deeper state of *samādhi,* a great ocean of consciousness arises when the meditator forgets the feeling of his body and he identifies himself with that eternal ocean of consciousness. At that state he feels "I am Brahman." This mental state, enlightened by concentration on *anāhata nādam* after complete relaxation, destroys his ignorance and doubt regarding universal consciousness. To obtain this state you must make strong mental suggestions: "I am Brahman." Repeat them until you get identity with supreme consciousness. After enthusiastic practice you will be successful in doing so.

3. *Ayamātmā Brahman.* After a few years' practice in actuality you will feel that your Self is really the part of the supreme Self, which is one-without-a-second. You will feel: "This Self is Brahman," "This entire universe is Brahman."

4. *Prajñānam Brahman.* The more concentration is advanced, the more consciousness, peace, bliss, and existence are advanced. Finally you will feel that the intuition and consciousness that were always with you and that gave you constant judgment for every good and evil activity are fully magnified in yourself, and now there is not the least difference between knowledge and the Self; you will perceive "Consciousness is Brahman."

5. *Satcidānandam Brahman.* Personality depends on the following three factors:

a. Existence
b. Understanding and knowledge
c. Peace and bliss

No living being can live without these factors. Personality develops with the development of these three and, on the other hand, personality decreases with the diminishing of them. For example, when one does something wrong or evil one endangers one's existence, understanding and knowledge become weak, and peace and bliss are in danger of being obliterated. Therefore, existence, knowledge, and peace constitute personality. Conditional existence, knowledge, and peace constitute conditional or individual personality. On the other hand, unconditional existence, knowledge, and peace constitute unconditional personality. In advanced meditation conditional existence, conditional understanding, and conditional peace are transformed into unconditional, eternal existence, understanding, and peace respectively.

In the deepest state of *samādhi* the entire universe is melted into an immeasurable ocean of consciousness and magnetism. The meditator experiences directly identity with the ocean of eternal consciousness. eternal knowledge, and eternal existence. This is the ultimate state of *param puruṣa* with *param śakti* (supreme consciousness with supreme energy and nature). This is the state of *jivan mukta.* At this point the meditator attains freedom.

1. Place your body in an easy posture.
2. Relax your entire body.
3. Practice to suspend your breath.
4. Mentally and firmly make the five suggestions.
5. Repeat the suggestions one after another, but do not repeat all during the same practice period. Each suggestion needs separate practice in the beginning.
6. Feel the electromagnetic pulsations in your entire body and in the entire atmosphere.
7. Feel that the consciousness which is in your body is the consciousness of the universe, and feel that life is an electrical phenomenon.
8. Feel that the natural elements of your body are the natural elements of the universal nature.
9. Feel the great ocean of consciousness and magnetism flowing in you and around you.
10. Feel that your body is magnetized completely and that it is the transmitter and receiver of your consciousness; you are not limited by your body.
11. Feel that you are everywhere.
12. Feel that innumerable suns, moons, stars, and planets are in you. They come and go, but you are the changeless eternal principle.
13. Concentrate your whole energy on *anāhata nādam,* and feel eternal consciousness, existence, peace, happiness, and bliss are manifested everywhere.
14. Wish for the welfare and happiness of all.
15. Think and feel that the entire universe is in you and you are in the entire universe.

16. Identify yourself with eternal existence, eternal consciousness, eternal peace.

This is the end of the twenty-third lesson. Read it, understand it. Enlarge it with your commentary. Concentrate on *śabda brahman* (*anāhata nādam*). Forget about your body and identify yourself with *Brahman* through these five great suggestions. When you obtain the state of eternal consciousness, eternal existence, and eternal peace and happiness, through *samādhi,* you will attain freedom and *nirvāṇam.*

24

ĀSANAS—POSTURES—OR DISCIPLINE OF THE BODY

The body and the mind are interdependent. The mind cannot function when the body is suffering from physical diseases, and the body is not normal when there are mental diseases. The science of Yoga psychology recognizes the importance of both of them. It prescribes exercises for both the body and the mind, so that they may develop themselves in a psychophysiological equilibrium, and they should produce complete co-operation to manifest Universal Consciousness and they should cease to enslave the Self. By practice of postures, consciousness becomes free from bondage and weakness, and realizes a boundless existence of infinite bliss. The body has as much dignity as the mind. Consciousness is manifested according to the development of the body and the mind; the body is the shadow of the mind.

Āsana, or posture, is a physical help for concentration. In the sleeping and agitated states, meditation is impossible. There are innumerable postures and it is impossible to describe them all. Here I will satisfy the beginner by giving the principles of postures and then I will leave everything for him to decide, selecting whichever posture he wants. The same posture cannot be recommended for everyone. The same posture is not always suitable for the same person at different times; therefore you should practice as many as possible. Postures must have the following qualities:

1. A posture should relax the body and the mind.

2. It should give strength to the body and the mind.
3. It should remove all mental and physical burdens, anxieties, and diseases.
4. A posture should help to forget the feeling of the body so that consciousness may identify itself with supreme consciousness.
5. A posture should give cultural and therapeutic advantages.
6. A posture should be uninterrupted, firm and easy. Painful postures should not be adopted for concentration.

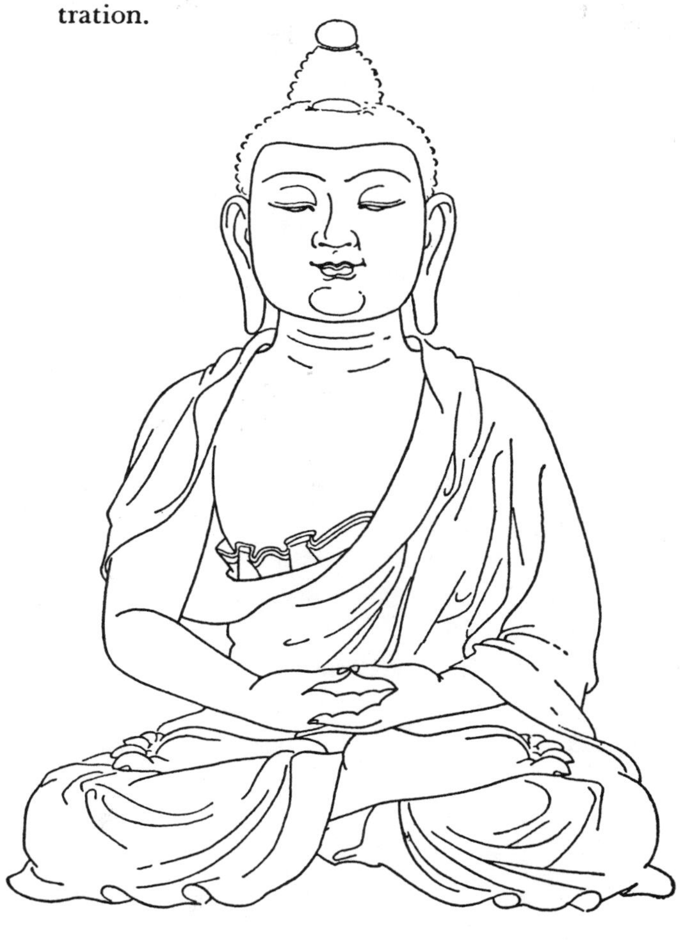

VII

MEDITATIVE POSTURE

Padmāsana . . . the Lotus Pose

Gives complete relaxation and equilibrium
Greater blood supply to pelvic region, benefiting coccygeal and sacral nerves
Enables yogi to contract and manipulate the abdominal muscles

Consult books or an expert on *Haṭha* Yoga and gradually practice difficult postures, but for concentration select as easy a posture as possible.

By the practice of postures, the body is led from animal incontinence to divine strength.

You should be careful about the food you eat. You should not eat and drink things that can cause disease in the body and make a sloth of it, cause the nerves to be on edge, stimulate the senses, etc. Lower desires always try to strangulate the higher desires and true joy of the spirit. Bodily needs must be subordinated to mental, moral, and spiritual development.

The later stages of Yoga demand great physical strength with endurance, and if the body is not trained through postures, *samādhi* will be impossible. A strenuous spiritual life strains the earthen vessel of the body to the breaking point; therefore the body must be brought under perfect control through discipline and exercises.

Haṭha Yoga trains the mind to sharpen the instrument of the body to remove the body's poisonous conditions. It trains it to remove fatigue and to arrest its tendency to decay and old age. The aim of Yoga is to control the body, and not to kill it, as some monks teach.

Perfection of the body consists of beauty, grace, strength, and adamantine hardness.

You do not require difficult postures for concentration. In the beginning select an easy posture, and add a daily 10-minute practice of a few difficult *Haṭha* Yoga postures. Thus, in a few months you will be able to perform all those postures which professional Yogis demonstrate. Be sure that the postures are a means to Yoga and concentration, and not the end of Yoga. Some people misunderstand postures as Yoga and philosophy. A man asked his wife what Yoga means. She replied: "Head down, legs up, eating vegetables, is called Yoga." Here she meant the postures of Yoga, but not the real Yoga. Some people think Yoga means yogurt.

When a recent critic of Indian culture assured his readers that Indian philosophers think that sitting cross-legged and contemplating one's navel are the best ways of sounding the depths of the universe, he had in mind one of the postures of *Haṭha* Yoga, shown at hotel and other lectures in Western countries.

VIII

ĀSANAS

Sarvāñgāsana . . . Shoulder Stand (*Left*)

Stimulates thyroid and improves health of entire body
Benefits age degenerated sex glands of both sexes, displaced uterus, etc.
Relieves dyspepsia, constipation, hernia and visceroptosis and benefits abdomen

Śīrśāsana . . . Head Stand (*Right*)

Sends increased blood supply to brain, pineal body and pituitary gland—

benefits cardiac and digestive systems
tones up the nervous system
helps remove headaches, dizziness, and arterio-sclerosis
improves intelligence and memory
treats the degeneration of nerve centers
benefits liver, spleen, sexual degeneration
hernia and visceroptosis treated
relieves asthmatic discomfort

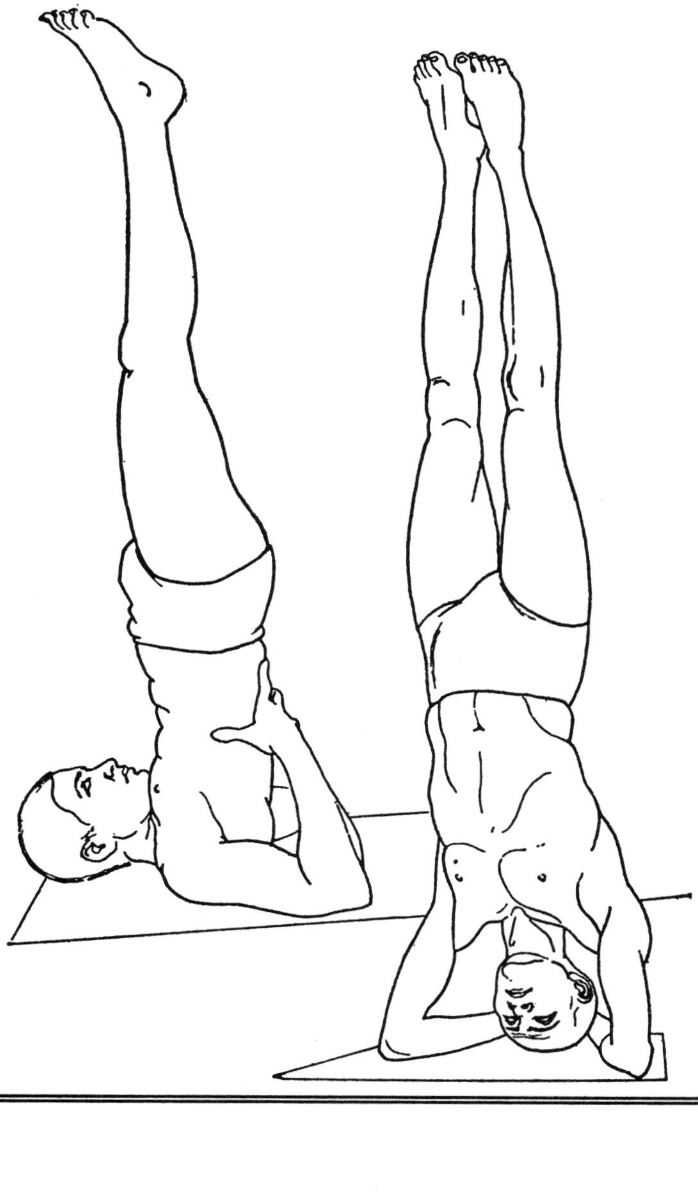

IX

ĀSANAS

Posture for Meditation and Complete Relaxation (*Top*)

Śavāsana . . . the Dead Body Pose (*Bottom*)

Relaxes body and mind
Soothes and rests nerves and muscles
Venous blood circulates to heart and fatigue is removed
Helps reduce high blood pressure
Alleviates nervous conditions

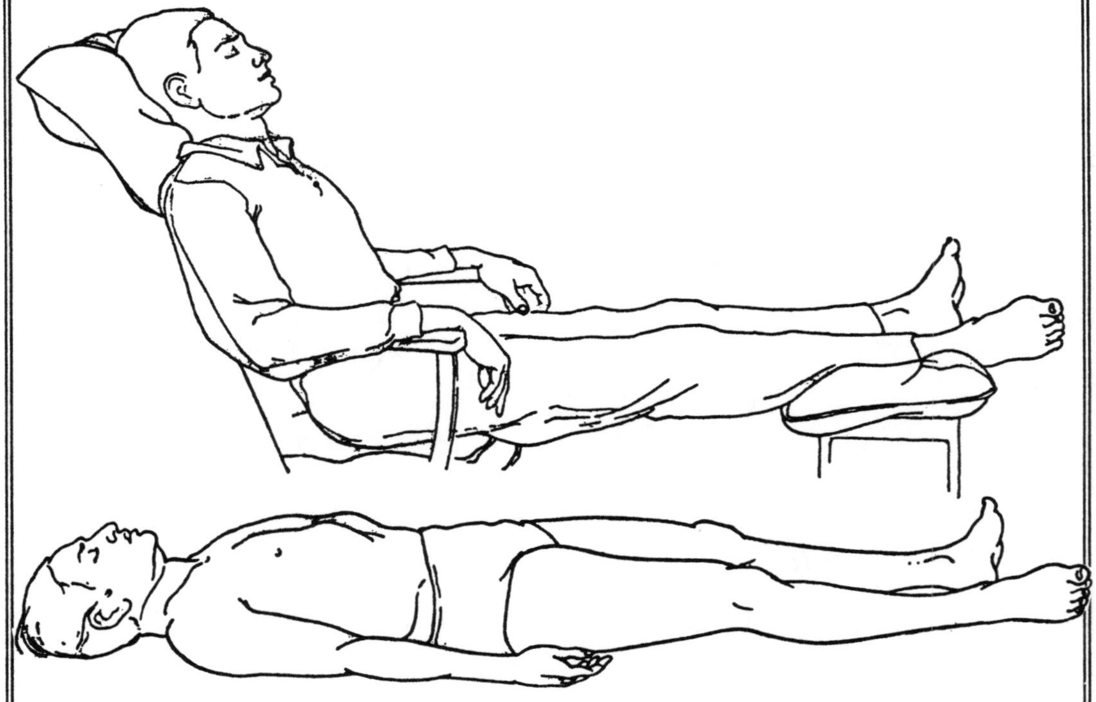

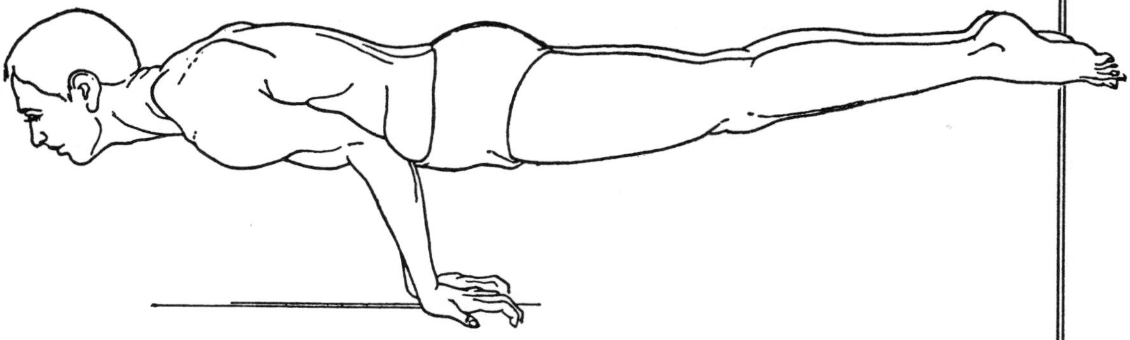

X

ĀSANAS

Mayūrāsana . . . Peacock Pose (*Top*)

Elbows pressing into abdomen and liver increases blood supply
removes chest and abdominal diseases
reduces abdominal fat, piles and constipation
helps evacuation of excretory system
brings perfect balance to the body

Halāsana . . . Plough Pose (*Bottom*)

Removes joint diseases
reduces abdominal and chest fat, strengthens muscles
renders the spine elastic
benefits the upright standing posture
also stimulates thyroid and health of entire body

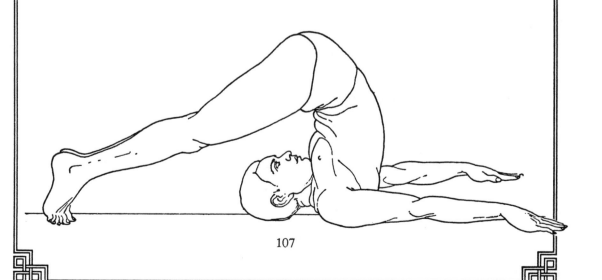

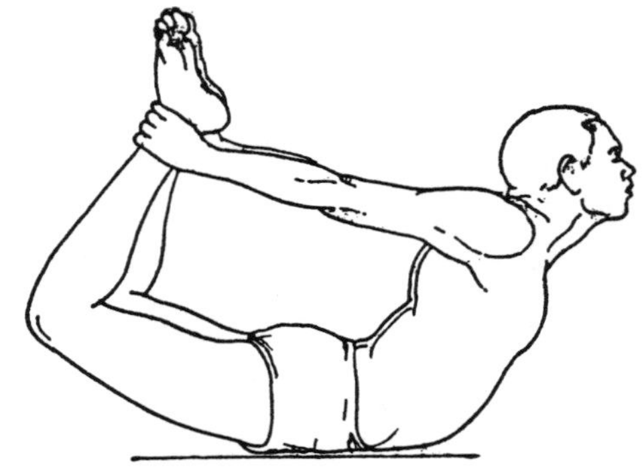

X I

ĀSANAS

Dhanurāsana . . . the Bow Pose (*Upper Left*)

Stretches muscles of abdomen and hips
Corrects spinal curvature tendencies
Alleviates stomach gas condition
Reduces abdominal fat

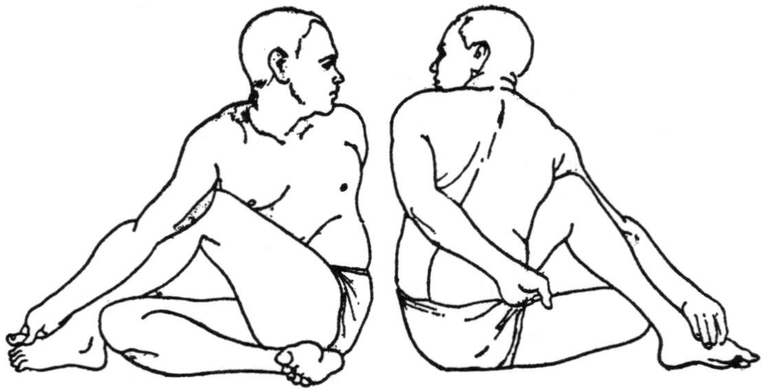

Ardha-matsyendrāsana . . . the Twist (*Upper Right*)

Twists the spine to the two sides
Spinal column and sympathetic nervous system benefited
Muscles of shoulders and abdomen are massaged
Constipation and dyspepsia are relieved
Good for the liver, spleen and kidneys

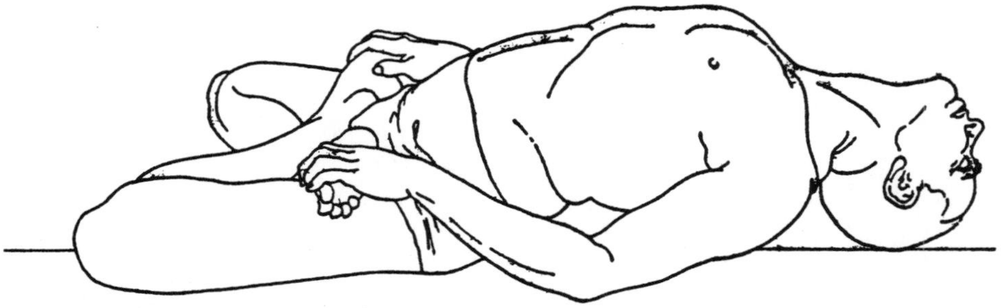

Matsyāsana . . . the Fish Pose (*Bottom*)

Benefits back, neck and chest
Can float in water for long periods in this pose
Arrests sexual and abdominal degeneration

XII
ĀSANAS

Bhūjaṃgāsana . . . the Cobra Pose (*Top*)

Strengthens back and abdominal muscles
Corrects displacement tendencies in spinal column
Benefits spinal column, parasympathetic and sympathetic nervous systems
Indigestion and flatulence are aided

Salabhāsana . . . the Locust Pose (*Bottom*)

Benefits pelvis and abdomen
Strengthens the back muscles
Aids circulation in the legs

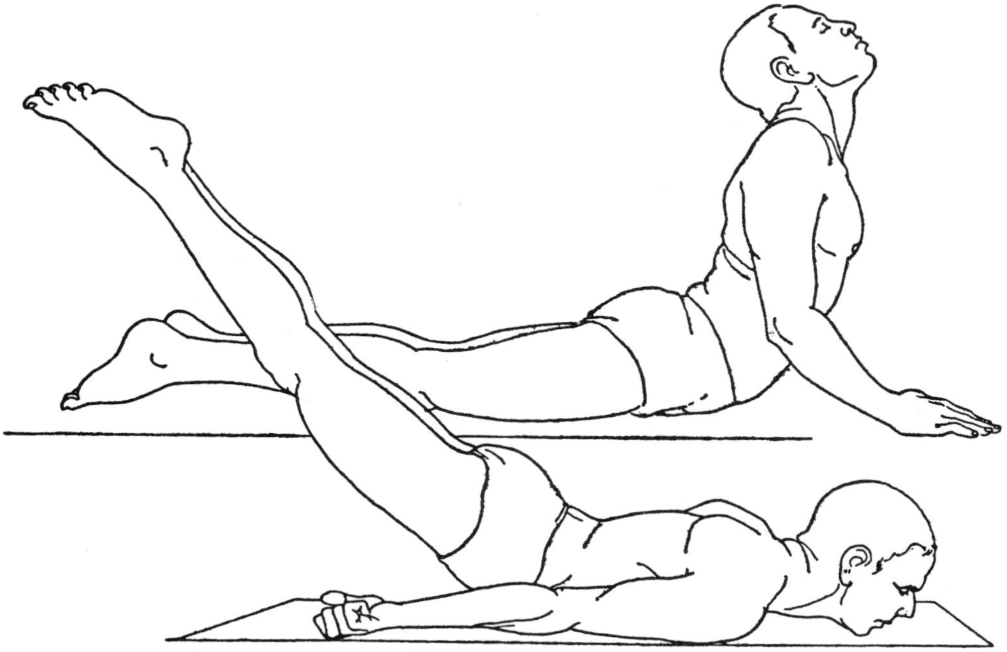

The aim of *āsanas* is to train the mind and body for spiritual perfection and not as mere physical exercises. Ninety-nine per cent of the books written on this subject are by inexperienced persons.

Every posture should give you spiritual uplift and electromagnetic pulsation in your body. I will leave this to you: to relax different parts and select different postures by which you can perceive magnetism soon, and can create *yoganidra* in your body.

This is the end of the twenty-fourth lesson. Read it. Consult an expert on *haṭha* Yoga. Read the right books on this subject. Practice gradually, and you will be able to perform all those postures which are performed by *Hatha* Yogis.

25

PRĀNA AND PRĀNĀYĀMA

General Description: The whole manifested universe is composed of two materials:

1. *Prāṇa* (primal energy).
2. *Ākāśa* (primordial nature).

Both are omnipresent, omnipotent, and all-penetrating existences. By the energy of *prāṇa, ākāśa* is manifested in this universe. Everything that is manifested, with or without form, with name or without name, is *ākāśa*. Air, liquids, solids, the sun, earth, moon, stars, organic bodies, and inorganic bodies, all are the manifestation of *ākāśa*. It is so subtle that it cannot be perceived by the physical senses. When it takes gross forms, then it is perceived by the physical senses. At the beginning of the manifestation, air, light, liquids, and the solid forms of matter are derived from *ākāśa,* and at the end of the cycle they all melt into *ākāśa* again and, thus, the cycle from and to *ākāśa* is going on perpetually.

As every material form is derived from *ākāśa,* so every form of energy is derived from *prāṇa*. All forces in the beginning of the cycle come out of *prāṇa,* and at the end of the cycle they resolve back into *prāṇa*. Force of motion, magnetism, gravitation, electricity, sound, heat, thought, etc., are examples of *prāṇa*. The sum total of all forces in the universe, mental and physical, when resolved back to the original state, is called *prāṇa*.

In short, supreme nature has two aspects: the nuclear

aspect and the aspect of energy. All the nuclear aspects of nature are the manifestation of *ākāśa,* and all forms of energy that reside within the nuclear state are from *prāṇa.*

As the nucleus and nuclear energy are not separate, so the *ākāśa* and *prāṇa* are inseparable. As nuclear energy is obtained from the nucleus with great effort by nuclear mechanisms, so also the energy of *prāṇa* is obtained from *ākāśa* with great effort through the perceptual mechanism, the psychic mechanism.

Prāṇāyāma means the *āyāma* (manifestation, expansion), or splitting of *ākāśa* into *prāṇa* or *prāṇas* (primal energy). By the process of *prāṇāyāma,* individual energy and consciousness are expanded into universal energy and consciousness, and because they are eternal, therefore one becomes eternal and immortal by obtaining that form. *Prāṇāyāma,* therefore, means control of universal *prāṇa.* Breathing exercise is not the whole of *prāṇāyāma,* as many people think, but it is only one of the many exercises through which one arrives at real *prāṇāyāma.* The whole concentration, meditation, and study of Self-analysis is *prāṇāyāma.*

Here we want to discuss breathing exercises that help us to reach the real *prāṇāyāma.* First we want to consider the nature of breathing.

Every living being is in the living state because it breathes. The moment it ceases to breathe, it is pronounced dead. There is no exception to this eternal law. Biological life and consciousness depend on breathing. Breathing is called respiration. Breathing of every living being consists of three states:

1. *Pūrakam:* The state of inhalation. By this process one fills one's lungs and cells with air.
2. *Kumbhakam:* The state of restraining. In this state there is an exchange of gaseous substance. Toxic air is replaced by fresh *prāṇa* in the tissues and the lungs.
3. *Recakam:* The state of exhalation. By this process all the toxic air and other toxic substances are removed from the chest.

The whole body is doing respiration, but the skin and lungs are the main systems of respiration. Therefore they constitute the chief respiratory system.

This whole respiration is divided into two main classes:

1. External Respiration: This consists of three phases: (a) Ventilation, (b) Gaseous Exchange, and (c) Circulation of *prāṇa.*
2. Internal Respiration: This consists of oxidation and other metabolic actions and reactions.

The body tissues, especially the nerve tissues, cannot live without oxygen, and this oxygen is part of *prāṇa,* which we breathe with every inspiration.

Food is taken through the alimentary canal. After primary digestion, chyle is sent to the heart and lungs. This chyle has food energy in potential form. Oxygen is mixed with this chyle in the lungs, and oxygenated blood is sent through circulation to every cell tissue of the body. Every cell tissue is a small factory which, with the help of oxygen, breaks down the potential energy of the food substance into actual energy. This actual energy is then used by the body for general development, and by the senses for the development of different sensations and understanding through them.

The process of cell division by new morphology, the exchange of carbon with oxygen and other foodstuffs, metabolism and oxidation, and organization of the cells into special groups, these and all other functions of the body depend on internal respiration. Thus *prāṇa,* which we take in through breathing, performs two types of respiration: external and internal.

Through breathing exercises we strengthen both respirations directly. One should do breathing exercises up to the point of exhaustion and perspiration; these are the signs of internal respiration. When perspiration and exhaustion start in the body, one should understand that internal respiration is stimulated, and one should stop breathing exercises at this point to give internal respiration a chance to operate fully.

In breathing exercises, with every expiration in succession, impurities of the body are removed through the lungs, skin, and kidneys, and with every inspiration in succession, universal energy, life, and light of knowledge are drawn into the body through the lungs and skin.

Energy of the sun operates freely in the body through conduction, convection, and radiation. The inner light continually increases until it reaches full freedom or salvation.

AFFERENT NERVE IMPULSES | EFFERENT NERVE IMPULSES

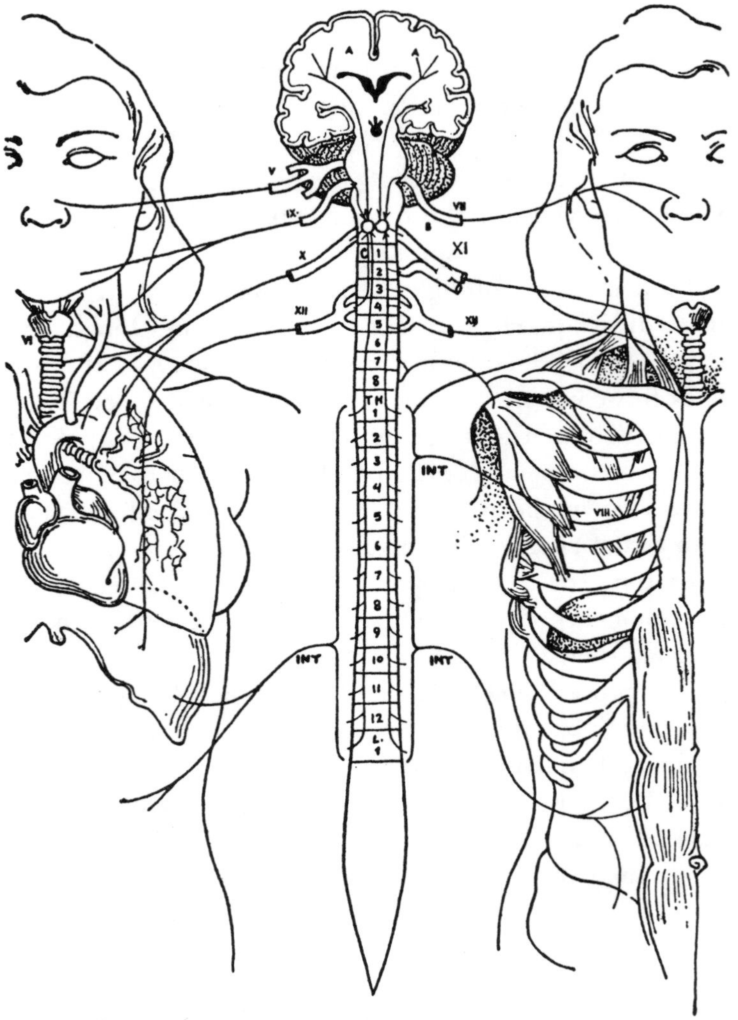

Courtesy, The CIBA Collection of Medical Illustrations

XIII

CONTROL OF RESPIRATION

A. Cortical Control over Medullary Center
B. Respiratory Center in Medulla

1–8 Cervical Nerves } All the nerves of the respiratory system
1–12 Thoracic Nerves }

v. Trigeminal Nerve
vi. Larynx and Trachea
vii. Facial Nerve
viii. Ribs and Muscles as part of Respiratory Mechanism
ix. Glossopharyngeal
x. Vagus
xi. Spinal Accessory
xii. Phrenic Nerve going to the Diaphragm

Just as the impurities of metals, such as gold, silver, etc., are destroyed by heating them in fire, similarly, mental and physical diseases and other defects of the body, the mind, and the senses are burned by the fire of *prāṇāyāma,* and their purity is achieved by the performance of breathing exercises. Just as a vacuum cleaner removes all kinds of dirt from the house, so the suction machine of breathing exercises sucks up all defects from the body, senses, and mind, and removes them through expiration, perspiration, and other excretory channels.

Definitions of Prāṇāyāma:

1. The state of concentration in which the movement of the heart for inspiration and expiration is stopped is called the perfect state of *prāṇāyāma;* one identifies one's self with supreme consciousness.
2. The state of concentration in which the movement of the chest for inspiration and expiration is forgotten and unknown to the meditator, and he identifies himself with supreme consciousness, is called advanced *prāṇāyāma.*
3. That state in which the respiratory system is trained by forcing air in and out is called the breathing exercise of *prāṇāyāma;* it leads gradually and ultimately to the above mentioned states.

The first two are components of *Rāja* Yoga and the latter is part of *Haṭha* Yoga. According to force and location of air, *prāṇāyāma* consists of the following four varieties.

1. *Bāhya vṛitti* (external forceful location of air).
2. *Abhyāntara vṛitti* (internal forceful location of air).
3. *Stumbha vṛitti* (immovable forceful control of air).
4. *Bāhya bhyāntara viśnayakṣepī* (multiple intake and output of air).

1. *Bāhya vṛitti* (external forceful location of air): Just as strong vomiting throws out food and water, similarly the breath should be forcibly thrown out and checked as long as possible. When you intend to expel the breath, the pelvis should be pulled upward, and kept up as long as the breath remains out. When there is a feeling of uneasiness and suffocation, then

the breath should be slowly drawn in. The above process should be repeated according to capacity and desire. The process should be accompanied by the recitation of OM mentally. This conduces to the purification and firmness of the body, senses, mind, and consciousness. This may be called external *prāṇāyāma.*

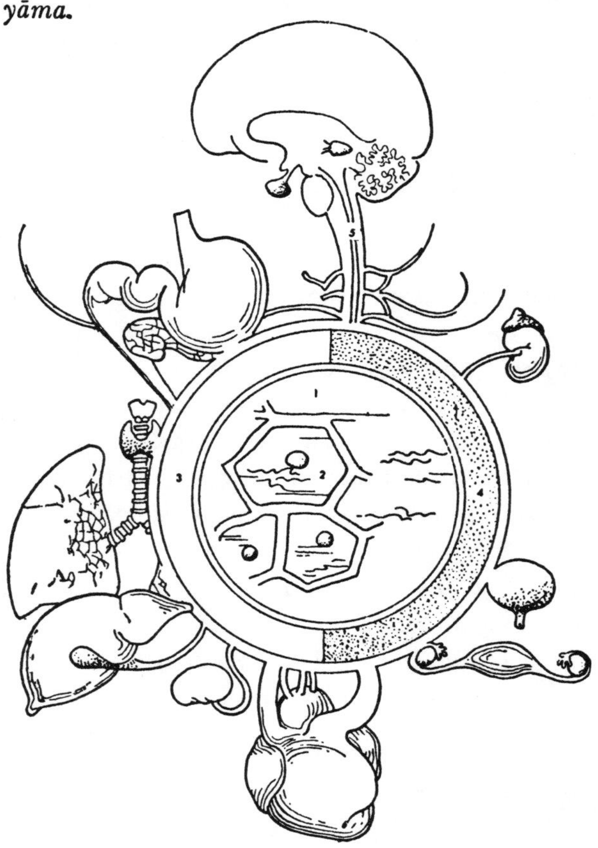

XIV

THE INTERNAL ENVIRONMENT

Life depends on internal fluid circulation: intra-cellular and interstitial fluids. This internal environment is constant, remaining the same in extreme cold or extreme heat. All endocrine glands, the digestive system, respiratory system, the liver and illustrated organs are constantly pouring their secretions and hormones into the internal environment through cardiac circulation. This whole environment is influenced by the mental faculty. The thinking process influences the entire system. In higher meditation the entire internal environment is influenced and the meditator heals all hidden and active diseases. This is the subtle nuclear system of treatment to reorganize the body as a whole.

1. Interstitial fluid
2. Intra-cellular fluid.
3. Venous blood
4. Arterial blood
5. Spinal fluid

2. *Abhyāntara vṛitti* (internal forceful location of air): The first *prāṇāyām* ends in the second. Inhaled breath is stopped inside as long as possible. Repetition of OM is similar to the first, and it ends in the first; that is to say, in expiration. Thus, expiration and its pause, and inspiration and its pause are repeated according to capacity. This makes one cycle of *prāṇāyāma,* which consists of the four above mentioned phases: a. expiration (and its) b. pause; c. inspiration (and its) d. pause.
3. *Stumbha vṛitti prāṇāyāma:* In this *prāṇāyāma,* air is neither taken in nor is it removed. It is immediate checking, i.e., stopping the air all at once, inside in and outside out. The chest remains like a straight pillar in a standstill position, or like a motionless jar full of liquid. Therefore, it is called *stumbha vṛitti prāṇāyāma* (*stumbha,* pillar; *vṛitti,* similar).
4. The fourth *prāṇāyāma* is out-in-holding *prāṇāyāma.* In this breathing exercise the air is drawn in deeply and held, and when it has a tendency to go out, forcibly another amount of air is taken. This is the first phase, the state of inspiration. The second phase is the state of expiration. Remove the air from the chest and when it has a tendency to return, exhale it forcibly again. The lungs have a surprising capacity for air. It is impossible to empty the lungs completely. Therefore, do not worry about the expulsion of air again and again. This is the state of counterreaction. By counterreacting on inspiration and expiration, both movements are kept in check, and the respiratory center in the medulla comes under control, which leads to the subjugation of the senses and the mind. This process increases strength and energy and so sharpens the intellect, which can easily comprehend even the most abstruse and subtle problems. This helps the development of the hormonal secretions, and *ojas śakti* (vital force) in the human body which, in turn, are productive of firm strength, courage, control of the senses, and acquisition of the knowledge of all sciences in no time.

The Principle of Prāṇāyāma. The entire body, house of the senses, mind, and consciousness, depends on *prāṇa.*

If in ordinary conditions the cerebral cortex is without air for five minutes, there will be total death. The body really cannot live without oxygen, even a single moment. Even during those five minutes it uses its internal oxygen. Thus, breathing is life. By the exercise of *prāṇāyāma,* the breathing is strengthened and, consequently, life is strengthened.

Prāṇa is the greatest force in the universe. All forces are nothing but its manifestations. When *prāṇa* is manifested in its full form, life is manifested in true form.

In breathing exercises, internal and external pressures come into friction and, consequently, they awaken the entire central nervous system, the body and senses. For instance, when air is removed, the internal pressure of the lungs and body is decreased and the atmospheric pressure operates forcefully on the whole body to stimulate every body tissue. When air is taken in, the internal pressure is increased and there is friction between external and internal pressure. Therefore, *prāṇāyāma* means the exercise of the internal and external pressure, which ultimately leads to the state of full control of breathing and perfection.

There is no method known to the world to check the restless mind and senses other than *prāṇāyāma.* It is the powerful engine to lead the mechanism of the body, senses, and mind to the state of perfection. As a rope tied to the feet of a bird can bring it down, so the exercise of *prāṇa* controls the restless mind and its waves. *Prāṇa* is the infallible electric rod to control the lion of lust, desire, and anger.

From the point of view of concentration and exercise, *prāṇāyāma* is classified as follows:

1. *Rāja Yoga prāṇāyāma*
2. *Haṭha Yoga prāṇāyāma*

The *Rāja* Yoga *prāṇāyāma* is carried out by will power only. The fingers are not used for these breathing exercises. In *Haṭha* Yoga *prāṇāyāma* the fingers of the right hand are divided into three groups. The right thumb is placed on the right nostril, the ring finger and little finger are placed on the left nostril, and the index and middle fingers are folded into the palm.

The beginning is found in the *Haṭha* Yoga *prāṇāyāma.* No one can perform *Rāja* Yoga *prāṇāyāma* without being an expert in *Haṭha* Yoga *prāṇāyāma.* In the state of *Rāja* Yoga, the entire body remains in the state of *yoganidra.* The entire body is as if dead; therefore the hands and fingers cannot work in that state. The mind is enlightened, and by the power of the mind breathing is stopped and *prāṇāyāma* is performed by the mind only.

Technique of the Haṭha Yoga Prāṇāyāma.

1. Place your body in such a comfortable posture that your chest, neck, and head are kept in a straight line.
2. Remove all anxieties and waves from your mind and be cheerful and happy, because in a restless state you cannot perform *prāṇāyāma* fully.
3. Press your right nostril tightly with your right thumb.
4. Inhale slowly through your left nostril. Fill your entire chest with air and remember that you are doing external and internal breathing exercises.
5. When you take air in, repeat OM mentally and think that you are carrying life from the external world to the internal world; that is to say, to every cell.
6. Think that you are removing all physical and mental diseases from your body.
7. When inhalation is complete, place your ring and little finger on your left nostril and press it tightly, This is called *kumbhakam.*
8. Restrain the breath as long as possible. Repeat OM.
9. When restraining becomes impossible and you feel uneasiness and suffocation, start exhalation slowly by lifting your right thumb from the right nostril.
10. After complete exhalation, now press your left nostril first with the ring and little finger of the right hand and inhale slowly through the right nostril. When inhalation is complete, press right nostril tightly with right thumb and restrain exhalation. When you cannot maintain the air within, exhale it through your left nostril by lifting your right ring and little finger from the left nostril. This is called one cycle of *prāṇāyāma.*

11. Repeat as many cycles as possible. Reach the point of exhaustion and perspiration, which are the manifestations of internal breathing.
12. Feel that your entire body is full of electromagnetic pulsation.
13. Feel that with every pulsation the heart is sending life and energy to every tissue of the body.
14. Feel that with every heartbeat your body is being magnetized and your mind is awakening.
15. When you are exhausted, stop the exercise and meditate in a relaxed position.
16. Listen attentively to *anāhata nādam.*
17. *Haṭha Yoga prāṇāyāma* ends in *rāja Yoga prāṇāyāma.* Regulate your breathing in the meditative state.
18. In this state, breathing should be as slow as possible.
19. In *rāja Yoga prāṇāyāma,* inhalation, restraining, and exhalation should be performed mentally.
20. When OM—*anāhata nādam*—is manifested in full form, forget the body, breathing, and everything.
21. Develop that habit so that you are not aware of your own breathing, in the same way as you do not know your breathing when you are solving any serious problem.
22. Continue this practice daily, eat moderately, and you will be successful in your *prāṇāyāma.*
23. Repeat OM chanting as long as possible. This is external *kumbhakam,* which gives you tremendous power and complete mental peace.
24. Chanting of OM should be begun at a low point and must reach up to the highest point of your voice.
25. When you are tired of chanting, meditate on OM.
26. Forget the feeling of the body and identify yourself with supreme consciousness.

Combination of Prāṇāyāma *with Relaxation.* When you relax any part of your body, fix your mind on that part, send strong suggestions to relax that part, and feel sensation of relaxation in that part. Hold your breath and feel electromagnetic pulsation in that part. For combined practice of *prāṇāyāma,* the body is divided into seven zones:

1. Control of sex organs with the control of *prāṇa.*

2. Relaxation of legs with the control of *prāṇa,* fixing it on the lower part of the spinal cord.
3. Relaxation of abdomen with the control of *prāṇa,* fixing it on the center of the abdomen (navel).
4. Relaxation of chest with the control of *prāṇa,* fixing it on the heart.
5. Relaxation of neck with the control of breath, fixing it on the neck.
6. Relaxation of the entire body by fixing attention and *prāṇa* to the place of the third eye and by holding the breath.
7. Complete identity with supreme consciousness by fixing *prāṇa* and attention on *sahasrāram* (cerebral cortex).

Now you know how to combine *prāṇa* to awaken *kuṇḍalinī* through the seven *cakras.*

Technique. Hold your breath and send your energy and power of attention from *mūlādhāra* to *sahasrāram* and from *sahasrāram* to *mūlādhāra* (lower part of spinal cord to cerebral cortex and from cerebral cortex to the lower part of the spinal cord). Repeat this process until you forget your body and identify yourself with supreme consciousness.

Practice *prāṇāyāma* daily. *Prāṇāyāma* will teach you *prāṇāyāma.* When breathing is held and you see the entire universe in you and yourself in the whole universe, this will be the highest state of *rāja Yoga prāṇāyāma.* Do not fear; this is the highest state of life, when a mortal becomes an immortal. When you obtain this state through *prāṇāyāma,* you will attain eternal life, existence, consciousness, and bliss. To go to any world or to take any form will be possible.

How Respiration is Centralized by Prāṇas *through Central Nervous System* (Suśumna).

1. Respiration is under voluntary control (cortical) and involuntary control (reflex).
2. It is regulated by integrated action of muscular, nervous, and chemical mechanisms.

3. The pace-maker is the respiratory center in the medulla.
4. It adjusts the source of supply (external respiration) to the needs of the body (internal respiration).
5. Inspiratory stimuli are received at the center in the medulla by afferent nerves and expiratory stimuli are transmitted by efferent nerves.
   a. *Muscular Mechanism:* The enlargement of the chest on inspiration exerts a suction pull on the lungs and as the lungs expand with the expansion of the chest, air flows into the lungs. Inspiration is the active component and expiration is the passive one. The chest, diaphragm, and abdominal muscles resume their previous position following the elastic recoil of the lungs. Chest muscles and diaphragm are the chief muscles used by the muscular mechanism.
   b. *Nervous Mechanism:* All those nerves that innervate the chest, abdominal muscles, and diaphragm directly form the nervous mechanism. Other spinal nerves support the nervous mechanism indirectly for breathing. Thus, all spinal nerves are engaged in respiration. From the lungs a succession of impulses is set up in the vagus nerve from stretched receptors of the vagus nerve in the lung tissues. The stimuli reach the respiratory center. The respiratory center in the medulla induces shortening of inspiration and initiates expiration. The receptors of the vagus nerve stretched in the heart, aorta, and carotid sinuses act as a result of both pressure and chemical changes in the blood. Increased arterial pressure induces reflex inhibition of the respiratory center. Lowering of the arterial pressure stimulates the center and causes hyperpnea. Increased venous pressure stimulates the center and causes hyperpnea and lowering venous pressure induces reflex inhibition of the respiratory center. Thus, venous pressure change is exactly the reverse of arterial pressure change. Pressosensitive nerve endings are situated mainly in the wall of the dilated portion of the internal carotid artery.
   c. *Chemical Mechanism:* Carbon dioxide and lactic

acid are the chief chemical regulators of respiration. They increase the hydrogen-ion concentration in the blood. An increase of the carbon dioxide content of the alveolar air of as little as 0.2 per cent stimulates increased respiratory effort by direct action on the respiratory center and also reflexly by stimulation of the sensory nerve endings in the carotid sinus region and aortic arch. Within fairly wide limits, ventilation is not influenced by the amount of oxygen inhaled. In rarefied atmosphere at high altitudes, where oxygen pressure in the air is greatly reduced, increased ventilatory effort is required to compensate for the lack of oxygen.

Summary. The respiratory center in the medulla receives stimuli from the higher cortical centers, which are controlled by psychic power, and it receives afferent (sensory) impulses by way of the trigeminal nerve (fifth cranial), glosso-pharyngeal nerve (ninth cranial), vagal (tenth cranial), phrenic nerve (from cervical segments 3, 4, 5), and lower intercostal nerves (from thoracic segments 1 to 12). Efferent impulses (motor) are transmitted by way of facial (seventh cranial), vagal or wandering (tenth cranial), accessory (eleventh cranial), phrenic (from cervical segments 3, 4, 5), cervical (from segments 1 to 8) and intercostal nerves (from thoracic segments 1 to 12).

Meditate on respiration through *nādam*. Direct the energy of *nādam* into the whole body through external and internal inspiration and remove the obstruction, excrement, defect, filth, ignorance from the body, senses, and the mind through internal and external expiration. Flow air in gently, and with the air flowing in, fill every portion of the body, senses, and mind with divine power through external and internal inspiration, and remove material desire, lust, anger, hatred, and demon nature out of the body, the senses, and the mind through internal and external respiration. Continue this process until *nādam* (OM vibration) becomes the nature of external and internal breathing. When *nādam* is in and out and breathing is regularly controlled, one feels oneself in the ocean of consciousness. One's consciousness is absorbed into supreme consciousness and one expands one's individual personality into Universal Personality.

Practice this meditation daily through the path of *kuṇḍalinī* and awaken your *kuṇḍalinī* power gradually. By awakening *kuṇḍalinī* power, obtain the true mental body, which is eternal and immortal.

This is the end of the twenty-fifth lesson. Read it, understand it. Consult charts of respiratory mechanism and the relation of the respiratory center to the entire body. Study the biochemistry of respiration. Concentrate with *prāṇa* and enjoy *nirvāṇam.*

26

THE AURA AND ASTRAL BODIES

Everyone is interested in opening his third eye, to awaken *kuṇḍalinī śakti* and to see the aura and astral bodies, but how many are ready to make the necessary sacrifices to achieve this? This particular lesson refers to the aura and astral bodies.

Introduction. Every element of Nature is full of auras and every living being has astral bodies. They are fully developed in the human being; even our shadows and photographs have auras.

Auras present innumerable colors; these colors are classified in the following manner: red, orange, yellow, green, blue, indigo, and violet.

The astral bodies are five in number; their first three forms are visible to adepts, and the two subtlest forms are visible only to those who are perfect in the practice of Yoga. The first form, which is called the physical body, is visible to everyone, and all the subtle bodies are manifested through this physical body. Their manifestation is in accordance with the development of the physical body. If the physical body is not pure, then the astral bodies, although ever manifested, are not visible to that particular soul which is incorporated in that body. At the time of death, these bodies are disconnected and are transmigrated to another incarnation. In the sleeping state these astral bodies can wander anywhere, but they are not disconnected from our physical bodies. Sometimes they are disconnected from the subconscious mind. Consequently, we are able to see the temporary death of such a person, and after a time we can see his resurrection. The explanation of resurrection is that apparently the body was disconnected, but actually it was still connected to the subconscious mind. These astral bodies can give information if they are visible through practice. They are visible after initial practice, but they cannot give the expected results to the beginner.

In our daily lives we obtain information from others, and can read others' minds through the astral bodies, but their working principle is unknown to the uninitiated. On the other hand, sometimes we misconstrue their message. If we develop our minds to read them properly, we can interpret their message exactly. All our ideas, images, and thoughts are the presentation of these bodies. Our dreams are presented by them; the bodies which we see in dreams are astral bodies, and the world presented in dreams is the astral world. Still, it is difficult for beginners to see them in the waking state.

Following is a brief method for developing the mind to see astral bodies and the aura:

First Method.

1. Stand before a full-length mirror in order to be able to see your entire body.
2. Practice *trāṭakam* constantly on your image in the mirror, without blinking. When your eyes are tired or strained, close them and meditate on your image as long as the eyes remain tired.
3. Repeat *trāṭakam.* In the beginning you can repeat *trāṭakam* four or five times. After long practice you will be able to see your astral body distinctly emanating from your body.

Second Method.

1. Place your body in a comfortable posture and practice *trāṭakam* with half-open eyes, without focusing on any particular object.
2. Within a few months' practice you will be able to see the aura of every object. You will see distinctly that everything is surrounded by an aura; even pictures and images. After a few years' practice you will be able to see astral bodies in your waking state.

Third Method.

1. Before falling asleep, give a strong suggestion to your subconscious mind: "I want to see my subtle or astral body." In the beginning you will not receive any reaction, but after a certain length of time you will feel a reaction from your subconscious mind, sometimes partially and sometimes completely. After making suggestions for a long time, you will be able to see your astral body and that of others while in the waking state.

Fourth Method.

1. Practice *trāṭakam* twice daily on the photograph of a liberated man. After a few days of faithful practice, you will be able to see light radiating from the picture, and after constant practice, you will be able to see distinctly your own astral body, as well as that of others.

General Description. Yoga psychology is entirely against these practices; they are merely the by-products of Yoga. Do not meditate nor concentrate for auras or astral bodies but meditate for perfection and liberation and, thanks to the grace of liberated souls, you will be able to see these and other supernatural phenomena.

For the student of Yoga a severe warning is given not to practice to see auras and astral bodies, because sometimes these practices cause degeneration of the mind. This lesson is written because some people are unbalanced and thus deviate from the right path. They practice Yoga only for this purpose, and therefore they misuse Yoga. Astral bodies and auras are very superficial things. If you practice in order to see them, it will require a good many years for you to see them, but if you do not practice to see them and practice Yoga in a right way, they will come before you after a few days' practice. On the other hand, this lesson will help you to familiarize yourself with the various manifestations and protect you from psychic fears; many students become bewildered by these psychic phenomena. If you are already familiar with the fact that these phenomena are in your way, you will not be frightened and you will be able to make good use of them.

Those who practice for astral bodies and auras as their principal aim spend their entire lives, and still these astral bodies do not serve their purpose. They are slaves to these phenomena and are always frightened by various psychic phenomena. Sometimes this practice may lead to spiritualism and, through spiritualism, it may create psychiatric problems. Therefore, students of Yoga should never practice for astral bodies and auras. They will appear during his practice, and he should understand at that time that they are coming to serve him. He should not pay any special attention to them. After a certain period of practice, he will feel that all astral bodies and other supernormal phenomena are completely under his command.

This is the end of the twenty-sixth lesson. Read it, understand it, and practice Yoga for perfection.

27

SUPERNATURAL POWERS

Definition. The powers not in the realm of unenlightened senses are called supernormal or supernatural powers. In the normal state, the range of senses is limited. Their field cannot go beyond their limit and cannot go below their limit. This limitation is called "Threshold of Instruments." Here, "instruments" mean senses and mind. But when, owing to certain practices, this threshold is removed or enlarged, one begins to acquire supernatural powers. Really, there is not such a thing as supernatural or supernormal power, because there is nothing beyond nature. This term is used, not from the point of view of nature, but from the viewpoint of man, his normal state, and his nature or capacity. Knowledge is the real power. When it is manifested beyond the limit of unenlightened man, it is called supernormal. This is really a relative term. Relatively, everyone has a few supernormal powers and qualities that are not found in others.

Supernatural powers are obtained by the following ways:

1. Birth: Sometimes a person had practiced Yoga in his previous incarnation, and in the present incarnation he is born with *siddhas* (powers).
2. Chemical Means: The modern world daily sees the miracles of chemistry.
3. *Mantram* and Study: Powers are obtained through

the learning of sciences and through the repetition of *mantras*.

4. *Tapaḥ:* Self-discipline and self-castigation.
5. *Samādhi* and concentration.

The supernatural powers obtained from the first four ways are secondary and temporary. *Samādhi* (concentration) is the means through which one can gain everything and anything, mental, moral, and spiritual. Supernatural powers derived through concentration are permanent and infinite.

There are innumerable varieties of supernatural powers, but here I will mention only those which beginners can understand and obtain through hard practice of concentration:

1. *Aveśa:* Entering into other bodies.
2. *Cetaśo jñānam:* Telepathy.
3. *Arthana chandataḥkriya:* Doing things according to one's own will.
4. Clairvoyance.
5. Clairaudience.
6. Omniscience.
7. Effulgence.
8. Vanishing from sight at will.

These eight are the sovereign powers of the Yogis. All these and other powers are obtained when the mind is pure through concentration and meditation. Be sure that all these attainments are perfections for the restless mind, and obstructions to *samādhi* if they are misused. Therefore, one must be careful not to misuse them because their misuse may lead to the world of name and form. Their proper use leads to perfection.

The acquisition of these powers is subordinated to the chief end of *samādhi* in the Yoga system. Though the highest goal may not be attained, the lower stages are not without their values. Each stage of concentration brings its own reward. Mastery in postures results in magnetizing the entire body so that it becomes hard and firm, able to tolerate the extremes of heat and cold, pain and pressure, and all other pairs of opposites. *Prāṇāyāma* removes all impurities from the mind, and the mind is enlightened with intuitive knowledge. *Saṃyamaḥ* gives perfect control of the body; mental and physical diseases are removed, and the mind becomes the abode of extrasensory perceptions. Through *saṃyamaḥ* (fixation, suggestion, and sensation) one knows the inmost cause of things and one reaches the great light of wisdom.

With the combination of *pratyāhāra* (withdrawal of energy and consciousness and their use for special purposes) and *saṃyamaḥ,* physical powers are increased and one has greater strength. By *saṃyamaḥ* and *pratyāhāra,* powers of the senses are heightened and one can hear and see at a distance. By long use of concentration, one can know one's past and future incarnations.

When *saṃyamaḥ* (fixation, suggestion, and sensation) is used on a presented idea, knowledge of another's mind arises. Transmission of thought from one individual to another, without the intervention of the normal communicating perceptual mechanism, is performed by students of Yoga.

Through *saṃyamaḥ* on the threefold modifications (manifestation, preservation, and dissolution) of nature, one obtains knowledge of the past, present, and future.

In the advanced state of Yoga, a Yogi can make his body invisible by the combination of *samyamah.* With the seven other steps of Yoga, one attains power to visit the entire cosmic space, the starry system, the polar star, and all other hidden scenes of nature unknown to the world.

Through concentration, he who discerns the distinction between the self and objective existence gains authority over all states of existence and omniscience. When one obtains them, they are regarded as perfection, but their misuse will be an obstacle to *samādhi,* which is the door of liberation. Therefore, one should not concentrate upon or hanker after supernatural powers. Do not worry, as they will come to you if you do not want them. If you want them, perhaps they may not come to you, or may come after long sacrifices. They are the by-product of Yoga. They are the flowers which one chances to pick on the road, but the true seeker does not go out of his way to gather them, because his principal aim is not only to pick up flowers, but to pick up fruit, which is freedom or emancipation. When all these perfections are utilized for the service of the supreme, then salvation can be obtained. He who falls victim to these supernatural powers rapidly goes downward and becomes part of the material world.

Supernatural powers are not occult, mysterious, or miraculous interferences with the laws of nature, but are part of that nature which is still beyond the senses of the unenlightened person. The world that is open to the unenlightened is part of nature but not the whole of nature. The world beyond the physical world has its own science and its own laws. The attraction of these powers indicates the higher life beyond the material life.

This is the end of the twenty-seventh lesson. Read it; understand it, and if any supernatural power comes to you, use it to enlighten your mind. Concentrate for perfection and not for powers. Do not be afraid or nervous when they come to you; they will not harm you.

28

ANĀHATA NĀDAM—OM—SPHOTAM

1. In the beginning was the Word, and the Word was with God, and the Word was God.
2. The same was in the beginning with God.
3. All things were made by Him; and without Him, was not anything made that was made.
4. In Him was life; and the life was the light of men.
5. And the light shineth in darkness, and the darkness comprehended it not.

Now you are familiar with the term OM and are in a position to begin concentrating on *nādam*. OM, *anāhata nādam,* and *sphotam* are synonymous. [This is called "Word" because of its derivation (Wor, *vara,* in Sanskrit, meaning truth, light, life; and D, to donate, to give;) that is to say, real life.] Everyone has this word but not everyone understands its real meaning. It shines in darkness, in ignorance; but owing to ignorance, man does not understand its omnipresent, omnipotent, and omniscient nature. It is the life and light of the universe.

A mighty ocean of *nādam* is flowing everywhere, in living beings and the nonliving, in the organic and the inorganic world, in manifest or unmanifest nature, in phenomenon or noumenon; in short, all states of nature and consciousness depend on OM. It is all in all, hence it is OM; it is all-powerful, almighty, therefore it is omnipotent; it is everywhere, therefore it is omnipresent; it knows everything and knowledge originates from it, therefore it is omniscient. There are a few synonyms for it, such as Amen, Omni, etc. They all have the same meaning.

You have the OM sound. Listen carefully to it. First you will hear it as a ringing sound in your ear, especially in your right ear. This is OM. It is called *anāhata nādam* because it is vibrating without instruments (*an,* not; *āhata,* instrument; *nādam,* sound).

There are two methods of listening to it: artificial and natural.

1. You can listen to this sound artificially by a *yogamudra* technique: Close your ears with your thumbs. Close your eyes with your index fingers. Close your nostrils with your middle fingers. Close and press together your upper and lower lips with your ring fingers and little fingers, respectively. The mouth should be filled with air, and breathe gently through the nose. By this *mudra* you will see the spectrum of different lights; you will hear *mantram* from your soul. This is a *yogamudra.* Through this *mudra,* you will see your soul in the shape of light and you will listen to its music in the form of *anāhata nādam.* If you see this light without obstruction for even a moment, you will be free from impurities and you will reach a higher stage.
2. When your impurities are removed up to a certain extent, you will begin to listen without placing your fingers on your face. This is called the real state of *nādam.*

NOTE: When you practice *yogamudra* and both of your nostrils are closed by your middle fingers, you will feel suffocation. To remove this suffocation, allow air through nostrils slowly and quietly, but do not remove your fingers from your nostrils. Do this daily for a few minutes and you will get real *anāhata nādam,* which will remain within you always and will teach you.

Anāhata nādam is the manifestation of the supreme into perceptual mechanism. When you have real *nādam,* meditate constantly on it. When all impurities of your mind are removed by meditating on OM, you will forget your physical, subtle, and causal bodies, and you will identify yourself with that eternal Self which is one-without-a-second. Practice it secretly; it will produce conviction at once. Ultimately it will transform you into the *nirvāṇa* state.

There are innumerable varieties of *nādam,* but they will be impractical for beginners. The following ten are the most useful and frequent:

1. *Cin nādam:* Like the hum of the honey-intoxicated bees; idling engine vibration; rainfall, whistling sounds; high frequency sound.
2. *Cincin nādam:* Waterfall, roaring of an ocean.
3. *Ghaṇṭa nādam:* Sound of a bell ringing.
4. *Śankha nādam:* Sound of a conch shell.
5. *Tantri vīṇa:* Nasal sound, humming sound like that of a wire string instrument.
6. *Tāla nādam:* Sound of a small tight drum.
7. *Venu nādam:* Sound of a flute.
8. *Mṛidaṃga:* Sound of a big bass drum.
9. *Bherī nādam:* Echoing sound.
10. *Megha nādam:* Roll of distant thunder.

These are ten states of *nādam,* and every state consists of innumerable varieties of sounds. By meditating on them, one destroys the ignorance of one's mind. When one fixes one's full attention on these eternal vibrations, being free from impurities, one achieves absorption into the supreme. When the mind of the meditator is exceedingly engaged in OM, he forgets the entire external world, including his own body and senses, and he identifies himself with OM in *samādhi.* By the practice of concentration on *nādam,* he gradually conquers all effects of the mind and *guṇas* (*rajoguṇa* and *tamoguṇa*) and he obtains the state of *brahman.*

Anāhata nādam is *śabda brahman, saguṇa brahman,* oversoul with supreme nature, and when OM is fully manifested it is called *nirguṇa brahman.*

As vibration is the cause of all sounds, so OM is the cause of all vibrations and motions, and because phenomenon and noumenon of nature are nothing but the vibrations and motions of the energy of nature, every state of nature is called the state of OM.

The macrocosm and the microcosm are passing through four states of OM. These states are classified according to the letters in OM. OM has four phases, three letters, and the fourth is the echo. All four states are called *nādam* or OM.

The letters of OM are: A - U - M, OM. The letter "A" in OM represents the manifestation and evolution of the microcosm and macrocosm; the consciousness of "A" which is operating in the microcosm is called *viśva,* and that of the macrocosm is called *virāt.* The letter "U" in OM represents the preservation of microcosm and macrocosm; conscious energy of "U," which is operating in the microcosm, is called *tejasā,* and that of the macrocosm is called *sūtrātman.* The letter "M" in OM represents the dissolution and involution of the microcosm and macrocosm; the conscious energy of "M" in the microcosm is called *prajñā,* and that of the macrocosm is called *īśvara.*

These three letters of OM represent three bodies and three states of existence of the microcosm and macrocosm. The letter "A" represents the gross body and waking state. The letter "U" represents the subtle body and dream state of existence. The letter "M" represents the causal body and the state of sound sleep, death, and the other unconscious states.

These letters consist of five sheaths, or *kośa* (coverings). The letter "A" consists of elemental *kośa.* The letter "U" consists of *manomaya, prāṇamaya,* and *vijñānamaya kośa:* sheath of the mind, *prāṇa,* and consciousness; sheath of the mind, life. The letter "M" consists of *ānand maya kośa,* (the sheath of bliss).

THE TABLE OF LETTERS OF OM

Letter	*Body*	*Conscious Energy*	*Sheath*	*State*
A	Gross	Universal *virāt* Individual *viśva*	*annamaya* Elemental	Waking
U	Subtle	Universal *sūtrātman* Individual *tejasā*	*manomaya prāna-maya vijñānamaya*	Dream
M	Causal	Universal *īśvara* Individual *prajñā*	*ānandamaya*	*suśupti* Sound sleep

This is the description of the letters in A - U - M, OM, but the vibrational part of OM or *nādam* is beyond description and beyond all these states mentioned above. Never has anyone been able to describe *nādam* fully. All the scriptures of the world describe it through indications. Therefore a full description of *nādam* means to put the infinite into the finite which is obviously not possible.

Examine your environment. In your room you see room atmosphere, space, and *ākāśa;* in your house, house atmosphere, space, and *ākāśa;* in your city, city atmosphere, space, and *ākāśa;* in the forest, forest atmosphere, space, and *ākāśa;* in the mountains, mountainous atmosphere, space, and *ākāśa;* in your country, country atmosphere, space, and *ākāśa;* on your planet, earth atmosphere, space, and *ākāśa.* But all these are parts of infinite atmosphere, space, and *ākāśa.* Likewise, *nādam* is infinite consciousness, of which the consciousnesses limited by the universal and individual elements are only parts and aspects. This pure consciousness is eternal, untouched by any limitation of manifested nature. The consciousness limited by the elements of universal and individual existence cannot exist without the infinite consciousness.

We have already mentioned three states of OM, such as the waking, dreaming, and sound sleep state. This state of *nādam* is beyond them; therefore, figuratively, it is called *turiya* (the fourth in number). It is transcendental consciousness, inexpressible in words and incomprehensible to the material mind, and it is the greatest of all. Therefore it is called *Brahman* (the greatest). It is beyond consciousness and unconsciousness, because in the biological sense these two states of existence have a limited meaning.

It is not that which is conscious of the internal world, nor that which is conscious of the external world, nor that which is conscious of both, nor that which is unconscious of both, nor that which is a mass of consciousness, nor that which is simple consciousness, nor that which is unconsciousness. It is unperceived by the sensory organs, incomprehensible by the material mind, unthinkable by thought, indescribable by tongue and pen, unrelated to any object, and it is uninferrable. It is the essential nature of the conscious and unconscious universe. It is the nucleus of the Self and the negation of all the phenomena of nature. It is eternal existence, eternal knowledge, eternal peace, eternal bliss, and one-without-a-second. This is called *nādam* and *turiya.* This is called *ātman* (Self) and you must realize it for your liberation.

It is not the fourth in numerical significance, but fourth in relation to the three states of consciousness, waking, dreaming, and sound sleep, which belong to the phenomenal world of nature. *Nādam* is the unrelated witness of the three states and, therefore, it is the absolute.

From the point of view of location, *nādam* is classified in four states:

1. The state of *nirvānam, parā* state. This is the highest state, which is one-without-a-second. Here, there is no distinction of subject and object. Only liberated Yogis can perceive it.
2. The state of *paśyanti.* In this state, supreme consciousness is fully manifested and the whole universe seems to melt into Universal *nādam.* The whole universe is filled with *nādam.*
3. *Madhyamā* state. When the whole body is filled with *nādam,* with the pulsation of the heart vibrating the surrounding atmosphere.
4. *Vaikharī state.* The manifestation of *nādam* in the head, especially in the ringing of the right ear. All letters are the manifestation of *vaikharī.*

The first state is infinite and eternal; the second state is universal; the third state is that of an advanced student of Yoga, and the fourth is that of beginners.

This is the end of the twenty-eighth lesson. Be sure that *nādam* is the foundation of concentration. Forget about your body, senses, and mind, and perceive the great ocean of *nādam* vibrating everywhere. Identify yourself with it, and you will be able to understand the significance of *samādhi.*

Before beginning the next lesson, on *samādhi,* repeat this chapter, understand it, and meditate on it.

NOTE: According to the development of meditation on *nādam* through the seven *cakras,* there are the following seven planes of consciousness:

Cakram	*Plane of Consciousness*
1. BHŪ	1. NĀDA MANIFEST

The all-pervading *nādam* is manifest in self-consciousness and the meditator listens as to some strange sound in his head.

2. BHUVAH	2. NĀDA COMMUNED

When one meditates on manifested *nādam* and its various developments, it is called "*Nāda*-communed." Here, the aspirant is absorbed in *nādam* temporarily, but only by his conscious effort. His meditation on *nādam* is neither unconscious as in the first, nor perpetual as in *samādhi,* but is dependent on his will power and the purity of the mind which leads his self-consciousness to the communion with *nādam*. Material attractions and irrelevant circumstances create frequent fluctuations in the mind. This is the state of initiation.

3. SWAHḤ — 3. NĀDA-MAD

In the eyes of the average man this is a lunatic state, but there is a wide gulf between the ordinary lunatic and the *nāda*-madman. The mind of the ordinary lunatic has failed to recognize the significance of the manifested world and has not prepared himself to answer the problems of the universe. He has degenerated into complete failure, and has fled into the realm of hallucination and delusion which are intolerable to society, because he wants to escape reality. A *nāda*-madman, to the contrary, has solved his problems and he does not care for those things which take him out of reality. His main aim is to escape unreality. This is why he is called *nāda*-mad. By increasing suggestion and by seeking contact with highly advanced Yogis and saints, one obtains this state. Here, by these contacts, his mind is so uplifted into the realm of reality that he does not want to come to the material plane. This state needs the constant presence of an expert master.

4. MAHAḤ — 4. NĀDA-ABSORBED

In this state one is continuously absorbed in *nādam* without any effort. The aspirant feels himself in the ocean of *nādam* like a sponge in the ocean. *Nādam* is in and around him. As a man breathes day and night, unaware of his breathing, so the aspirant experiences *nādam* without any conscious effort. As in an abnormal atmosphere man becomes aware of his breathing and goes back into normal breathing after conquering the situation, so the aspirant, due to undesirable and unfavorable situations and discussion, makes a conscious effort to listen to *nādam* but goes back to his *nāda*-absorbed state when the situation is cleared.

5. JANAḤ — 5. NĀDA-INTOXICATED

Intoxication by alcohol or drugs gives a sensation of well-being as long as the intoxicant is in sufficient concentration in the tissues. The drug-intoxicated feels happy and feels temporarily beyond cause-effect, space and time. But this is temporary intoxication, and in the long run it ruins health and deforms the body; it destroys natural beauty, degenerates organs and nerves and obliterates the mind, and eventually it leads the drunkard to a mental asylum. When alcohol or drug intoxication passes away the drunkard goes into the state of a so-called "hangover." The *nāda*-intoxicated man is in the permanent intoxication of *nādam* and remains permanently beyond cause-effect, space and time. Here intoxication is continual, ever-increasing, never decreasing. The body is rejuvenated, consciousness is awakened and mind is enlightened. Intoxication is unalloyed in nature, reviviscent in power and permanent in extension (time).

6. TAPAH | **6. NĀDA-MERGED**

When sugar or salt is mixed with water their components are ionized and they go into complete dissolution and make a homogeneous mixture. So, also, when self-consciousness is dissociated from the material plane and associated with universal *nādam,* it is *nāda*-merged. The limited "I," individual personality, is utterly annihilated and is united with infinite bliss, infinite power and infinite knowledge. One forgets consciousness and finite universe, including family, friends, body, etc. and is simply conscious of self as *nādam.*

7. SATYAM | **7. NIRVĀNAM OR NĀDA IDENTIFIED**

While in the sixth plane there is permanent union with reality, in the seventh plane there is permanent identity with reality. The Yogi is not only united with reality but he *is* reality. He is not only united with *Brahman,* but he *is Brahman.* As a fine wire in an electric bulb is identified with electric current and gives light to the world, so in the seventh plane of consciousness is self-consciousness identified with the electricity of *nādam (Brahman)* and enlightens the mind of the Yogi. As the sun enlightens the entire solar system so the enlightened person in the seventh plane of *nādam* has the capacity to enlighten the entire world. So he is called the World Enlightened One when he reaches this plane.

29

SAMĀDHI

Definition. When concentration reaches its climax, that highest point which restricts all fluctuations and wanderings of the mind and which liberates the Self to attain its real form is called *samādhi* (*sam,* completely; *ā,* entirely and forever; *dhi,* intuition). Literally, *samādhi* means the full manifestation of eternal and divine intuition.

Introduction. Samādhi is the prestate of *nirvāṇam* and ends in *nirvāṇam.* When it is fully manifested (Yoga insists on attaining freedom through *samādhi*) it is called *Yoga-samādhi.* In the ecstatic state of *samādhi,* the connections of the body, senses, and mind with the outer world are broken, and the inner world of the Self is opened. It lifts the soul from its temporal, mortal, finite, conditioned, changing, and imperfect existence into an eternal, immortal, unconditioned, infinite, permanent, and perfect life. The Self is liberated and attains to *nirvāṇam,* the eternal status.

General Description. There are two classes of *samādhi:*

1. *Samprajñāta:* Synonym *savikalpaka samādhi.*
2. *Asamprajñāta:* Synonym *nirvikalpaka samādhi.*

Samprajñāta Samādhi (*enlightenment, the superconscious state of the mind*): In *samprajñāta samādhi,* fixation, suggestion, and sensation (*dhāraṇā, dhyāna,* and *samādhi*) reach their climax. The body is fully magnetized, the senses go into the state of *yoganidra,* the mind is enlightened, and the Self is awakened from its long sleep (ignorance). The body gets tremendous power to tolerate the pairs of opposites, such as pain and pressure, touch and temperature, heat and cold, etc. The literal meaning of *samprajñāta* (*sam,* complete; *pra,* excelled, eternal; *ñāta,* knowledge) means full manifestation of eternal and divine intuition. This is the superconscious state of the mind. In this state, the mind stuff (*cittam*) is fully concentrated on consciousness, single in intent, and fully illumines the real form of the objective and subjective world.

Samprajñāta samādhi is the state of union with supreme consciousness. Here, knower, known, and process of knowing are manifested in full form. This is the triune junction and combination of three rivers, the Ganga, the Yamuna, and the Saraswati (knowledge, *karma,* and *bhakti*). In *samprajñāta samādhi,* one knows the object, not in the way of physiology and psychology, but one knows it because one is it. The thought and the object of thought are united here and, therefore, they are the same. Here is the perfection of *dhāraṇā, dhyāna,* and *samādhi* (fixation, suggestion, and sensation).

Samprajñāta samādhi consists of four states of thought:

1. Power of Reasoning and Questioning: When this state of thought dawns in the mind, one reasons everything and questions everything. In another way, this is the state of curiosity—curiosity about one's own existence, about the world around one's self, such as the sun, moon, earth, stars, planets, etc. Remember that curiosity is the mother of knowledge. If you do not know something, it simply indicates that you have no curiosity about that object. Curiosity will govern your mind twenty-four hours a day. In sleep you will have dreams about the object of your curiosity. It will remain in your mind as long as you do not know the real answer to that object. The curiosity of *samādhi* is not individual, but universal, because it has curiosity to know everything. Therefore, it takes a long time for the complete answer and perfection. This state ends in the second; that is to say, the power of knowledge.
2. The Power of Knowledge: When you are truly curious to know something, you will acquire knowledge about it. The power of knowledge gives the real an-

swer to curiosity, and the mind becomes full of knowledge. And because knowledge is the greatest power in the world, it is called the Power of Knowledge. By the power of knowledge and discrimination, you will be able to know truth and untruth; reality and unreality; purity and impurity; immortality and mortality; righteousness and unrighteousness; pleasure and pain; knowledge and ignorance; the Self and the nonself; light and darkness, etc. By knowing them, you will begin to mold your life in the light of the first in the pair and you will renounce the second. When the second in the pair, that is to say, impurity, unrighteousness, etc., are removed from your life, happiness and peace will dawn in the mind. The second state of thought ends in the third, the state of happiness.

3. The Power of Peace and Happiness: There are innumerable forms of peace and happiness. They are all manifestations of the Self. All material states that give peace and happiness are like the moon, because they reflect the light of the Self; but the Self is the source and the sun of the eternal light of peace and happiness. When the sun rises, electric lights, moonlight, etc., fade away. In the same way, when spiritual peace and happiness dawn in the mind, all material peace and happiness fade away before it.

   The power of peace and happiness is the real step to concentration because, when the mind is restless, concentration and meditation are impossible. Peace and happiness are the end of material life because all living beings live for peace and happiness. The real cause of suicide emerges when there is no hope of peace and happiness in the present or future life. While the material life ends in peace and happiness, the spiritual life starts from that very point; therefore, the peace and happiness of a spiritual person are impossible to describe. The third state of thought ends in the fourth.

4. The Power of Identity: Identity is the inherent power of the mind. While the body has the nature of union, the mind has the inherent tendency of identity. For instance, when we shake hands with someone, or dress ourselves, the body goes into union with the hands

and clothes, but when we study science, art, or any other learning, the mind identifies itseif with those studies. Union can be removed at any time, but identity is permanent. We can take off and put on clcthes, but the same relation does not exist with identity.

Schools, colleges, and all our teachings depend on the power of identity of the mind. Students in schools and colleges identify their minds daily with their respective subjects, and in due course they become experts in the identity of the mind. All degrees and diplomas are the results of identity.

When someone has the intention of lust and other material desires, he does not feel separation from his desires and lust, but he feels that he desires them. When one does meritorious work and consequently has illumination of the mind, he does not feel separation from that state, but he feels that he is illumined. The reason is simple. This feeling is due to the power of identity, which is the inherent nature of the mind.

Although it is an eternal fact without exception, people do not understand this psychological principle. The fourth state of *samprajñāta samādhi* fully refines the mind to obtain the full manifestation of identity. In the ordinary state, the mind has identified itself with matter; therefore it is called material mind, but in *samprajñāta samādhi* it identifies itself with the supreme; therefore it is called the Self and the Spirit.

Technique. There are two ways to concentrate: Active and passive. The active way begins with *dhāraṇā, dhyāna,* and *samādhi* (fixation, suggestion, and sensation), and the principal aim is the control of the external and internal nature of body, senses, and mind, meditating on *nādam.*

In the passive way, body, senses, and mind are forgotten completely, and absorption in the ocean of *nādam* is the main aim.

In the active way of concentration, a knowledge of anatomy, physiology, and Yoga psychology is necessary, because without knowledge of the seven *cakras, kuṇḍalinī,* and *suśumna,* active or positive concentration is impossible. Passive or negative concentration is the theme of *asam-*

prajñāta samādhi, where only consciousness is left and the entire universe is melted into it. In fact, there is no such thing as active, positive, or passive, negative concentration, but from a practical point of view this classification is extremely necessary. Without mastering positive concentration, negative concentration will be difficult if not impossible.

Beginners do not know "what is mind," "what is Universal Consciousness," and "what is the Self," but they know their body, senses, thinking, and individual consciousness. Therefore this is called positive concentration, these being known to them. Concentration on the Supreme is imaginary in the beginning, hence it is unknown and called the negative method. In fact, in later states the positive becomes negative, and the negative becomes positive, when the entire universe, including one's own body, is melted into it.

Technique of Samprajñāta Samādhi.

1. Regulate your diet. Eat simple food.
2. Remember, mentally, *yamas* and *niyamas.*
3. Select a strictly private place, and place your body so that it cannot fall. An easy chair would be excellent for Western people.
4. Practice *dhāraṇā, dhyāna,* and *samādhi* (fixation, suggestion, and sensation) on *nādam.*
5. Fix your mind on the entire *suśumna* (central nervous system) and send suggestions to the whole body through *kuṇḍalinī* (entire nervous system). Be careful to feel changes and sensations occurring in the conscious field.
6. Hold breath. Inspiration and expiration should be very regular and slow. They should not distract your attention from *samādhi.* If you find it too difficult, forget completely about the breathing; after enough practicing respiration will be regular. Sometimes it may even seem to stop. This state will bring an experience of great pleasure.
7. Practice general *pratyāhāra* as long as your body is not magnetized by the power of *yoganidra* and your mind is not enlightened.
8. By *pratyāhāra,* you will forget your body and feel an ocean of consciousness, light, and life around you

and within yourself. You will hardly believe that you have a body and that you are limited within a body.

9. Relax the entire body and think "I have no particular body, I am in every body."
10. Do not be afraid of this state. New awarenesses will come to help you and not to disturb you.
11. Sit in your meditation, not like a nervous person, but like a person who has faith, courage, and dignity.
12. The idea of death and of the body falling can disturb your entire process. Do not worry about death; this is only fear. No one has ever died in concentration on *nādam*.
13. Conquer fear of the body falling and of death. When fearlessness governs your consciousness, death will flee from you, and you will perceive the supreme Self shining like a trillion suns, collectively, radiating through the entire universe by its mighty primal energy, cooling your heart like innumerable moons, collectively, and giving you a message of liberation.
14. Your remaining *karmas* will be washed away. Your eyes will be filled with constant tears, and immediately you will perceive that you have complete identity with supreme consciousness and supreme nature.
15. Your face will radiate with aura and light, and you will remain in this ecstatic state for a long time after concentration. You will hardly believe that you have a body. In theism, it is called God-intoxication. You will see the entire world as though it were a dream.

    This is the supreme state of consciousness, and all supernatural powers will come to bless you. Do not pay any attention to them if you wish perfection in *samādhi*. Use all supernatural powers to understand nature and consciousness. They will open a new universe for your study. Use them but don't misuse them.

This is called *samprajñāta samādhi*. In this state you have supernatural powers but you still have all the impressions of material enjoyment in your mind. From time to time they will make a serious nuclear attack on you. If you are not careful, you may leave your practice and may fall from this high throne of the heavenly kingdom. These impressions work like demons and *śatan;* your own nature seems against you. Be careful to control this demon. Take complete refuge in *nādam.* Forget everything but *nādam* and control it.

Do not harbor a sense of pride because of your victory, because pride will disturb your entire victory. Victory is not due to your effort, but because of *nādam.* Be grateful to the supreme for your victory, and if you have failure, examine your methods carefully and be certain not to repeat the same mistakes in your life.

Impressions are still in the mind; therefore this *samādhi* is called *sabīja samādhi,* the *samādhi* in which the seeds of *karmas* and desires are still present. If you work carefully, you will conquer all difficulties.

This is a brief method of *samprajñāta samādhi* for beginners. There are innumerable other methods. You will know them all as you advance in your practice. This method will remain in your mind as your guidance.

The intuition obtained through *samādhi* is separate from the knowledge derived through sense perception, inference, and scriptural testimony, because this intuition is all-pervading, all-penetrating, and gives the power of omniscience, omnipresence, and omnipotence to the Yogi. Its object is concrete reality and not merely a general notion. It has power to transform object into subject, by which the Yogi knows the object in the closest way. The *satva* of *buddhi,* the essence of which is light (*prakāśa*), when freed from obscuration by impurity, begins to project constantly a steady pellucid flow of intuition which is not dominated by *rājas* and *tāmas* in *samādhi.* When this superreflective state of *samādhi* arises, the Yogin gains inner calm (*adhyātma prasāda*) and a mighty magnetic current of *sphotam* (*nādam*). By the power of this intuition, whatever you say and predict comes true; therefore it is called truth-bearing intuition (*ritambhāra prajñā*). Here is not even a trace of misconception.

In gross perception the senses perceive the object with the help of consciousness; therefore this perception is limited, mediate, and colored by the senses, but by the intuition of *samādhi* consciousness directly penetrates the objects, and the senses have ceased to work; therefore this perception is direct and immediate. In other words, all knowledge and sciences are the result of sensory perception, while *prajñā* (intuition of *samādhi*) is the result of extrasensory perception. Therefore, it is called "higher perception" (*param pratyakṣam*). It is seeing with the soul, while the physical eyes are closed. Once this intuition arises, its impressions and visions rule out all other impressions.

The experience of *samādhi* is inexpressible. One has no consciousness of body, senses, or mind. One knows that one has what one desired. One has obtained that state of consciousness where no deception can come, and one would never be willing to exchange one's bliss for anything.

In all organic and inorganic beings, there dwells a marvelous secret power of freeing every being, of withdrawing the Self from material life, and of discovering the eternal in every being in the form of unchangeability. The human body has especial privilege to this power. All the scriptures are but recorded experiences of seekers. Manifestation of the Self into Self is the exclusive experience of *samādhi,* upon which depends everything that you know of the supernatural and supersensual world. This experience of *samādhi* shows the seeker for the first time what real existence is, while all else only appears to be real. It differs from every presentation of the senses in its perfect freedom, while all other presentations are bound and overweighted by the burden of object. This experience occurs when one controls one's body, senses, and mind; forgets them fully and identifies one's Self with the supreme Self. At this stage the seeker annihilates time and space; he is no longer in time, but time and eternity are in him. This experience is not the personal property of any country or any man; it is universal. Anybody and everybody can feel it if ready to see it. It gives the greatest enjoyment and immortality, and it requires the greatest sacrifice When this state comes to the mind, man forgets everything and feels happy. In material life, this state is called sound sleep, which removes physical and mental fatigue, worries, etc., and gives physical and mental power; and in spiritual life it is called *nirvāṇam,* which gives liberation and spiritual power. Here is no room for personal pronouns, such as "I," "you," "he," "she," "it," etc. It is but what it is. Only practice will give you the real answer to this question. The scriptures and recorded experiences are only to inspire you; they are a guide to "it."

Asamprajñāta samādhi is the subject of passive or negative concentration; that is to say, it is obtained by the power of the spirit only, which is represented as infinite and negative power. Here, fixation, suggestion, and sensation are the external part of concentration. They are not an internal part of *asamprajñāta samādhi.*

In *asamprajñāta samādhi* a Yogi becomes like a motionless ocean. This is divine madness and the source of all powers in the universe. This is the highest and deepest state of happiness, peace, and blessing where intuitions are revealed in their perfect form.

Every soul is potentially divine and has eternal existence, knowledge, and bliss in potential form. Owing to the wanderings of the mind, it has lost its glory and the power of omniscience, omnipotence, and omnipresence. Immortal is suffering from mortality; infinite has become finite. Owing to the severe discipline of *asamprajñāta samādhi,* ignorance is destroyed, the infinite nature of the soul is revealed, and it gains its power of omniscience, omnipresence, and omnipotence. When the external and internal nature of the mind is controlled by *samādhi,* the soul's divinity is manifested in its full form. Visions and voices are regarded in Yoga as the superficial state of concentration, of materialism and mortality. This is a brief introduction of *samprajñāta samādhi,* and you will achieve it if you practice.

Asamprajñāta Samādhi. *Samādhi* is not a simple experience. It is infinite and inexpressible. It is a succession of mental states that grow more and more diverse and spiritual until they end in the *asamprajñāta* state of *samādhi. Asamprajñāta samādhi* means complete annihilation forever of dualism (not *samprajñāta,* knowledge of duality). This is the state that is called *nirvāṇam,* one-without-a-second. Here, there is no separate feeling of mind and matter, Self and nonself, consciousness and unconsciousness. This is such a positive experience that all experiences are submerged in it. This is such a great ocean of eternity that the entire universe is like salt to it; salt goes to measure the ocean but never comes back. The mind enters this state of *samādhi* but never comes back to its material state again. Here is no Self and no nonself. It is a wonderful experience, inexpressible by tongue or pen. This is the *anātm vāda* of Buddhism and complete self-surrender of theism. We cannot say that it is God, because God is a relative term that has no meaning without the universe, but here there is no universe. We cannot say it is the Self because the term Self has no meaning without nonself, but here there is no nonself. This is neither God nor non-God; neither Self nor nonself; neither consciousness nor unconsciousness. This is the state which is "all in all," omnipotent, omniscient, and omnipresent.

Asamprajñāta is that concentration where all material impressions are annihilated from the mind and, without mental waves, the mind returns to its own glory. This is the state that gives eternal peace and happiness.

Everyone has this state, whether he knows it or not. where a beginner receives them as the revelation of the creative spirit within himself. *Samprajñāta* and *asamprajñāta samādhi* are the highest states of enlightenment, when one not only gets vision, but also becomes vision; that is to say, union and identification with the supreme is the result of these two *samādhis,* respectively. And because the description of supreme consciousness and supreme nature are beyond tongue and pen, hence these two *samādhis* are beyond description. This is the subject of the mind. The mind has seen it but, unfortunately, has no tongue to speak about it, and the tongue has the power of speech but, alas, it has never seen it. Do not judge their authenticity by philosophy, reason, logic, and the other sciences, but go into practice and perceive them. They are waiting for you. They are judged by the light of practice. Philosophy starts from the point where physics ends, and *samādhi* starts from the point where philosophy ends. The end of physics is the beginning of metaphysics or philosophy, and the end of metaphysics is the beginning of *Yoga-samādhi.* Yoga does not recognize physics which is without metaphysics, and vice versa, metaphysics which is without physics. *Yoga-samādhi* is the beautiful bridge to cross the ocean of death, disease, and suffering, where physics and metaphysics work like a protective side pillar without which perhaps the vehicle of concentration may fall into the ocean of death through either side.

Asamprajñāta samādhi has two main classifications:

1. Mastery of the physical world (*bhāva pratyaya*). In this class the Yogin gets mastery over the physical world with his spiritual power, but if he neglects the power of the spirit and begins to play with the physical world, or if he does not have highest detachment and does not practice, he may fall from that state into the physical world again. In this state there is only partial liberation.

2. *Upāya pratyaya.* Mastery over individual consciousness and mind by the power of Universal Consciousness is obtained by developing the following methods:
   a. Highest degree of detachment from worldly things.
   b. Tremendous confidence in mental and spiritual power.
   c. Highest degree of energy and enthusiasm for the practice of *samādhi.*
   d. Mindfulness, constant memory of spiritual power.
   e. Development of the power of discrimination through the highest degree of intuition. By this power one sees things as they really are.
   f. Highest degree of devotion for one's teacher and the supreme (*nādam*).
   g. Honor and love for all living beings.
   h. Constant practice of *samādhi.*

These few means are mentioned here for the development of the *asamprajñāta* state. There are innumerable means; you can use them according to your situation and necessity.

Both of these states of *asamprajñāta* may be stated in the following way:

1. If you control the entire universe through the power of mind, it is called *bhāva pratyaya.* Here everything is controlled except the mind. Consequently, there are possibilities of coming down again.
2. By the power of the mind the full and perfect control of the mind is called *upāya pratyaya samādhi.* Here you do not need to control the entire universe separately because the universe is but a partial manifestation of the mind.

Upāya pratyaya asamprajñāta samādhi is called *nirvāṇam.* This is the highest and ultimate aim of human life.

Techniques of Asamprajñāta Samādhi. Remember the passive method of concentration, which means the control of self by the power of the self, or control of individual consciousness by the power of supreme consciousness:

1. Place your body in a suitable posture so that it will not fall over.
2. Master first *samprajñāta samādhi.*
3. Forget your body, your name, and your individual existence.
4. Constantly think: "I am *Brahman.* I am the supreme. The entire universe is the supreme. I am unborn and eternal. I have no death. I am eternity. I am peace (*śivoham*). I am eternal existence, knowledge, and bliss. I manifest the universe, I protect the universe, and I am the cause of the dissolution of the universe. Innumerable solar systems are manifested by me. I am operating through all bodies. I have no mortal senses, no mortal body, and no mortal soul and mind. I am deathless and birthless. All inorganic and organic beings are my form. I have no individual body, individual senses, individual mind, and individual soul. The entire universe is a waking dream. There is nothing except *Brahman. Brahman* is one-without-a-second and has eternal existence, knowledge, and bliss, and I am that."
5. "I have no death nor fear, nor any distinction of caste, creed, color, nor country; neither father nor mother, nor husband nor wife, nor children, neither friend nor enemy. I am eternal awareness. I am *Shiva,* I am *Shiva.*"

These are a few methods of *asamprajñāta samādhi.* When you practice *asamprajñāta samādhi,* you will find innumerable ways in the course of your practice.

Comparison between the *samprajñāta* and *asamprajñāta* states of *samādhi:* Concentration on the supreme through the analysis and synthesis of the universe and mind is part of *samprajñāta samādhi,* and concentration on *Brahman* through the power of *Brahman* is part of *asamprajñāta samādhi. Samprajñāta samādhi* is positive concentration, and *asamprajñāta samādhi* is negative. *Samprajñāta samādhi* still has the seed of future birth, and *asamprajñāta samādhi* has no future birth. In *samprajñāta samādhi,* birth and death are controlled by nature; and in *asamprajñāta samādhi* the liberated self has full freedom to take incarnation in any form. The Self has full freedom to do anything. *Sabīja samādhi* (*samādhi* with latent *karmas*), which gives the greatest power of understanding, is used as a stepping-stone to *nirvīja samādhi* (*asamprajñāta samādhi, samādhi* which conquers all *karmas*).

In *samprajñāta samādhi* residual potencies remain, but in *asamprajñāta samādhi* all residual impressions are destroyed. *Samprajñāta samādhi* is union with God, but *asamprajñāta samādhi* is to become God.

Until you reach the state of *samādhi,* your effort is the negative one for liberation. When, by the power of discrimination, the distinct nature of *puruṣa* (Consciousness) from *prakṛiti* is realized, the positive nature of spirit manifests itself. This manifestation of supreme consciousness on its own plane, above all confusion with *prakṛiti* (nature) is the highest state of *samādhi.* All possibility of confusion has ceased forever. An adequate description of *samādhi* cannot be written by pen, because the moment we open our mouth to speak, or hold a pen to write, we are not there. This is like a swimmer at the bottom of the ocean. As long as he is there, he cannot express his enjoyment, but when he comes up on the surface to express his enjoyment, he is not at the bottom. *Samprajñāta samādhi* is like swimming on the surface of the ocean, but *asamprajñāta samādhi* is like swimming at the bottom of the ocean of consciousness.

Know Yoga through Yoga. Yoga becomes manifest through Yoga.

He who is earnest about Yoga rests in it forever.

Samādhi is a state that few can attain, and almost none can possess for long, because it is broken by the calls of life. So it is said that final liberation is not possible without the special favor of the supreme teacher.

This is the end of the twenty-ninth and last lesson. Read it, understand it, and practice it.

30
OUR DAILY BUSINESS AND YOGA

Is it possible to obtain personal and business success through Yoga and *samādhi*? This is a great, puzzling, and baffling question that requires serious attention. There are many answers to this question. Some say that Yoga *samādhi* is not possible in the modern age, especially in congested cities. It is their opinion that it is only possible when it is practiced in a secluded country-like area. Others are of the opinion that one should renounce everything, including wife, husband, children, property, and business to become successful in Yoga. Some philosophers are of the opinion that Yoga is a supraethical system and therefore impossible for a common man.

We want to examine critically these and other like questions regarding the practice of Yoga, because if it is not possible to attain personal and business success through Yoga, then it will be part-time amusement and a matter of luxury, which will not require or deserve serious attention.

Before answering these questions, first we wish to discuss the meaning of "personal success" and "business success" and their far-reaching consequences. If personal and business success means to cut the throats of others, hypnotizing them by falsely sweet and polite conversation, as people generally do now-a-days, and to fill one's own treasure chest without paying favorable attention to others, then, really, Yoga is not the right instrument for them. If they have decided not to correct themselves or, on the contrary, they are considering Yoga as a divine instrument for material hoarding, then it would be advisable to leave the practice of Yoga as soon as possible.

Yoga is not the renunciation of personal life and business, but the renunciation of the vicious concepts parading as vital to these expressions. Personal life, business, marriage, and creation of children are part of the divine life. Therefore, they are not a hindrance in Yoga; but if they are not used as a part of divine life and are made the expression of animal life only, then, really, Yoga is against such a union. Yoga teaches the supraethical state of life, but that is the way leading to perfection. For beginners it teaches the practical way to concentrate the mind, which is the frame and skeleton of ethical and moral science. By this practice of Yoga, one reaches gradually that highest state of life which is beyond the capacity of common man and, therefore, it is called the superethical way of life.

The young, the old, the scientist, the layman, in short, anyone can practice Yoga. The practice of Yoga can be done in any place, provided that place is suitably soothing and peaceful. Yoga presents only one condition for concentration and that is calmness. Anything that is conducive to peacefulness of mind is necessary for Yoga, because without such a state of mind meditation is impossible.

If you really wish to become successful in your personal life and business or in any walk of life, concentration of the mind through the teachings of Yoga must be understood and mastered. Learn the power of influencing your own subconscious mind and in a short time you will wonder at the changes that will take place in your mental and physical development, and you will begin to notice that others are positively influenced by your personality. Courtesy and honest policies will enhance your business if based on truth. Truth is the foundation of ideal business. No doubt some people act as though they wish to be deceived; they seem not to believe the truth when it is not embellished. But you should not renounce truth to satisfy such persons. Business is of the greatest service for national and international development. However, it has two aspects: destructive and constructive. Misused, it destroys the individual, society, national and international relations; but if it is used as a divine source as well as practically, it is constructive.

You should behave with your business associates and clients as you would with your own family. Their welfare is your welfare. This is the secret of good business. You must truly feel good will in all your relationships; thus, your mind will be happy and your business will reflect this attitude day by day. To make mistakes or to do wrong in business is not new to the mind. It is common and not a crime if you are ready to learn right methods and to correct yourself. Mindfulness is a powerful force. It is called the waking suggestion. If you practice waking suggestions, you will improve yourself and your work capacities. At some time you may seem compelled to do wrong; it seems as though you cannot help yourself, as though you are being forced into wrong. The answer then is simple: your conscious mind is not alert. You become too lazy to correct yourself and become indifferent to the seriousness of your conduct. Thus, your conscious mind becomes negative to waking suggestions and you lose the positive power of the

The first two steps of Yoga, *yama* and *niyama,* intention to control mental powers and rules to materialize that intention—establish the foundation of Yoga practice. You should practice *ahiṃsā* (noninjury and nonviolence, truthfulness, honesty, protection of hormonal and vital powers of the body through continence, and reject the intention of hoarding money for selfish desires). It is not the bank account that creates trouble, but the mental programs and attitudes that seem unconcerned with the need to serve others. Money should be preserved carefully to serve yourself and society and to maintain national and international mind; and thus you create trouble for yourself and for your fellow human beings. By conducting your affairs without this consciousness you sow the seeds for further disorder in your immediate life and in the broader world around you.

You have within yourself a wireless mental telegraphy, a mental broadcasting station. Through this medium you broadcast your thoughts; therefore you should never transmit evil thoughts. By doing so you destroy not only your own welfare, but that of your fellow man, be he client or associate. Everything revolves in a circle; nothing runs in a straight line. Whatever you transfer comes back to you to make a complete circle. Without coming back to you, there will be no completion of the circle, and if this circle is completed by evil thoughts, destruction is certain. To be successful in thought transference, you must become very conscious of your own mental powerhouse, and you must

understand that the same mental voltage and will power are contained in other subconscious minds. You must use this power daily because without it your happiness may be destroyed. Yoga teaches you to be able to accomplish your aim through the positive use of this power.
welfare. If the bank account is utilized for personal use only (although legally you are free so to use it) from the viewpoint of Yoga this is the greatest sin. Modern political restlessness and wars are examples of this false philosophy. If one enjoys and ninety-nine suffer, we cannot establish a really democratic state. In short, we should not hoard for ourselves, injure anybody, should not practice untruth, theft, incontinence, or avarice. The chief virtue is *ahiṃsā,* and all other virtues are ruled by it. It is not only noninjury and nonviolence, but nonhatred. Abstinence from malice toward all living beings in every way and at all times is called *ahiṃsā.* Noninjury, truthfulness, nonstealing, continence and nonhoarding of money for personal satisfaction: these five are called *yamas.* The man who intends to control the mind and achieve fulfillment must follow the five *yamas.* This is called intention to control the mind and mental waves.

Cleanliness, contentment, austerity, study of Yoga scriptures and medium formation of one's own body is called *niyamas.* If one observes the *niyamas,* one materializes one's intention to control the mind and strengthen mental power. The following are four ways to create peace and happiness of the mind:

1. Friendship and fellowship with those who are liberated, because they know real happiness.
2. Sympathy and compassion for those who are suffering from mental and physical diseases or from any other circumstance.
3. Cheerfulness and gladness with those who are good, virtuous, and righteous.
4. Imperturbability and indifference to those who are evil minded.

These four methods, if made part of one's life, produce serenity (*citta prasādanam*). One should be free from jealousy and hatred, and should not be callous to the sufferings of other persons or nations. Hate sin but behave gently with sinners.

The principles of Yoga are absolute in their character and without exception. "Do not kill" is a categorical command of Yoga. We must not think of killing even those who may be against us, blasphemers, renegades of religions or government. The *yamas* and *niyamas* are of universal validity and have no exception of caste, creed, color, country, age, and condition. The persons who wish to be part of the higher life of meditation and concentration must follow them without fail.

For your success you must remember these two points: if you are not successful in any walk of life, first, do not worry, but second, follow carefully these two divine instruments:

1. *Practice:* It consists of:
   a. Long, constant efforts for concentration.
   b. Regularity of life.
   c. Great love and great confidence.
   d. Firm determination for practice.
2. Vairāgyam: *Nonattachment and Renunciation.* Renunciation does not mean to renounce family, home, country, social, national, and international life and to go to a forest or mountain for practice of concentration, but it means the removal of drawbacks, deficiencies, and those mental habits which are obstacles to higher life and concentration. Darkness and light, night and day cannot stand together. Bad habits and evil propensities are like darkness and night. One must renounce them for the sake of higher attainment. If renunciation means to renounce family, home, country, and society and to become beggars, monks, *swāmis,* then everybody will be wretched, and beggars and robbers will rule the world; maintenance of the welfare of the world would be impossible. This so-called renunciation is only a change of climate but it is not true renunciation.

Renunciation means the removal of mental weakness and drawbacks. If you have not firmly decided to correct your mind, then even the renunciation of the entire world will not help you. If world renunciation is regarded as renunciation, then death will be the only result, but fortunately this is not the case. Everybody tries to conquer death.

There is a great difference between change of climate and renunciation. No doubt change of climate helps if it is done properly, but one should not forget that one has one's mind with one's Self, and one has to refine one's mind.

No one can entirely renounce the primary necessities of life, such as food, clothes, accommodation, etc. Whether one is a monk or monkey, *swāmi* or beggar, one needs to fulfill one's primary necessities. Therefore, one should be careful to understand the meaning of renunciation. If one creates a troublesome atmosphere in the home, country, and society, and because of that trouble one renounces the world and takes refuge in the mountains, here perhaps the mountains can protect one from social and national punishment, but it is not renunciation. There is great confusion in understanding renunciation.

Renunciation is the secret weapon of Yoga and it is a succession of mental developments. The more we get light in practice, the more we renounce our weakness. Renunciation is proportional to our concentration, and one understands it step by step until one is able to remove the entire material covering from one's mind.

For renunciation of evil propensities and bad habits one should follow the methods given below:

1. *Pratipakṣa bhāvanam:* Think opposite forces against evil forces.
2. Loud pronunciation of OM.
3. Breathing exercises, especially holding of the breath.
4. Fasting, careful examination of diet, behavior, and company.
5. Keep busy, study everything that extends your understanding.
6. Consideration of the world as a waking dream.
7. Read the history of liberated men.
8. Exercise *pratyāhāra* on different parts of the body.
9. Meditate on effulgent supreme light, which is beyond all sorrows.
10. Consultation with teacher.
11. *Brahman bhāvanam:* Identification with supreme consciousness and complete forgetfulness of the body.

A stream of consciousness flows from the mind in both directions, toward construction and toward destruction, like rivers near the ocean. When it flows toward construction it attains freedom, knowledge, virtue and power, and when it runs toward destruction and nondiscrimination it begets ignorance, bondage, and weakness.

One attains twofold power of mind by renouncing one's weakness and evil habits.

1. *Apara vairāgyam:* First degree of renunciation. It consists of the renunciation of all material desires from the mind to attain mental powers. It brings purification of all business, systems, customs, and behaviors. One becomes master of one's body, senses, and mind. Lower and destructive desires cannot perturb one's calm nature. One's consciousness is awakened in this state to identify it with the supreme.
2. *Para vairāgyam:* Last degree of renunciation. It gives power to control entire nature and natural forces. This state brings mastery of nature. Here one attains full freedom and one is called an enlightened one. This state brings identification with the supreme.

Always remember that renunciation means removal of evil habits and shortcomings of life, because without renouncing them, you cannot truly develop your personality. This rule is without exception, whether in business, study, or any other field.

Be attentive toward impulse and compulsion. These are involuntary forces operating in your mind. These forces are of your own mind but now they are out of your control. By practice and renunciation you can control them and use them to develop your will power. Impulsion is a force from within and compulsion is a force from without. Where do these forces operate? In your subconscious mind, implanted by thought transference by you. These are your mental broadcasting stations. If you control them, your mind will be above the threshold of the world.

This is the end of the thirtieth chapter. It may at first be difficult for you to understand and grasp many of the facts written in it. But there are so many strange things in this universe that you will better understand after practice and study. Practice makes master and renunciation makes the nature of the spirit shine.

Read this book, understand it, and enlarge it a thousand times by your own commentary; practice it to become successful in your profession, business, customs, and behavior.

Yoga is the foundation of the ethical and moral life upon which the Kingdom of Heaven is established.

REVIEW

In accordance with the request of my students and friends, I have given here a brief introduction of ultimate reality, *nirvāṇam,* and full and complete instructions on every necessary point to ensure success of Self-realization through concentration of the mind and mental waves. I decided to make this course elementary and brief, and have done so in accordance with my promise to my friends. The lessons are so few and so simple that you may easily practice concentration in your home. If you practice the methods contained herein you will surely achieve success. I know that many of my students and friends have been successful with these methods. They have been tested and proved by innumerable liberated souls over a long period of time.

1. Never doubt your ability to control your mind.
2. Be positive that you have eternal existence, knowledge, and bliss.
3. Always observe silence, according to your leisure, and make powerful *dhāraṇā, dhyāna,* and *samādhi* (fixation, suggestion, and sensation).
4. Follow instructions given in each lesson.
5. Never become excited when you are in an unfavorable situation.
6. Never say "I will try to concentrate my mind," but say "I will control my mind. I will concentrate."
7. Do not become discouraged in your failure. You will eventually be successful in your practice.
8. Be sure that you can do anything and everything—whatever has been done by any liberated souls. Have

full confidence in yourself.

9. Understand exactly the science and psychology of Yoga to become successful.

Following is a review of the eight steps:

1. Make a firm determination to control your mind. This is the first step or *yama.*
2. Follow strict rules to accomplish your determination. This is the second step or *niyama.*
3. Place your body in a firm and steady posture. This is the third step, or *āsana.*
4. Practice control of your breathing. This is the fourth step, or *prānāyāma.*
5. Withdraw your conscious energy from the external world and external contact and identify yourself with supreme consciousness. This is the fifth step, or *pratyāhāra.*
6. Fix your mind for local concentration on particular *cakras* and limbs which you choose, and for general concentration on the entire body. This is the sixth step, or *dhārana* (fixation).
7. Send strong suggestion after fixation. The suggestion depends on your intention, whatever you want, such as anesthesia, cold like ice, hot like fire, and so on and so forth. This is the seventh step, or *dhyāna* (suggestion).
8. Feel sensation of your given order, whether your subconscious mind is able to follow your command or not. After due practice it will follow your order. This is the eighth step, or *samādhi* (sensation).

When you are firmly established to feel vivid currents of supreme consciousness in yourself and around you, you will attain unity of the supreme. You will feel the universe in yourself, and yourself in the entire universe. This is called *samprajñāta samādhi.* Ultimately this unity will end in identity with the supreme and you will feel that "that art thou." This is called *asamprajñāta samādhi* and will lead to final liberation.

The last three steps, *dhāraṇā, dhyāna,* and *samādhi* (fixation, suggestion, and sensation), are the internal components of *samprajñāta samādhi,* while the previous five are external components, or preliminary steps of Yoga.

In the state of *asamprajñāta samādhi,* the last three—*dhāraṇā, dhyāna,* and *samādhi* (fixation, suggestion, and sensation) also become an external part of practice, because this is the state of complete identity with the supreme. There is nothing beyond it. This is the state called one-without-a-second. Fixation, suggestion, and sensation belong to the world of dualism. Here is no dualism so they become external components of *asamprajñāta samādhi,* because they lead the consciousness up to the gateway of *asamprajñāta samādhi.*

My sincere desire is to make you successful in Self-realization through the concentration of mental powers. Whatever methods I obtained from my teacher, the world-enlightened one, *Bhagawāndās Bodhisatva,* I have published here briefly without any hesitation or reservation. When you are established in these practices, you will be the master of your mind and this mastery will open a new eternal and happy world for you. To obtain enlightenment, perfection, and freedom, study these methods, prove them. This extensive universe perceived by our senses is only the one-fourth part of that universe which is hidden in the divine plane. The other three-fourths part of the divine universe is strange and very little understood by the average person. A discovery of the eternal and immortal world is certain if you practice faithfully.

If you combine these methods with your practice, study, and experiences, you will obtain great confidence in mental power, conquer your obstacles, and attain full freedom in the realm of the spirit. Success is a by-product of practice. The whole universe will be your book. Books alone will not answer your curiosity. Practice these methods and obtain *nirvāṇam.*

OM

APPENDIX: ADDITIONAL ASANAS (YOGA POSTURES)

All Yoga postures and exercises are therapeutic in the following ways:

1. Promoting physical, mental, and spiritual beauty
2. Aiding meditation
3. Bringing about relaxation—physically, mentally, and spiritually
4. Preventing multiple sclerosis and other diseases of the nervous system
5. Preventing nervousness
6. Encouraging weight reduction
7. Stimulating breathing and circulation of blood and electricity in the whole body
8. Creating elasticity of the skeletal and muscular systems, and benefiting bones, muscles, and joints
9. Preventing stress and strain
10. Creating sound sleep and harmony with inner and outer atmosphere

Sūrya Namaskāra
Salutation to the Sun I - XII

Attunement to solar energy; to create elasticity of skeletal and muscular systems; for prevention of M.S.; for weight reduction, etc.

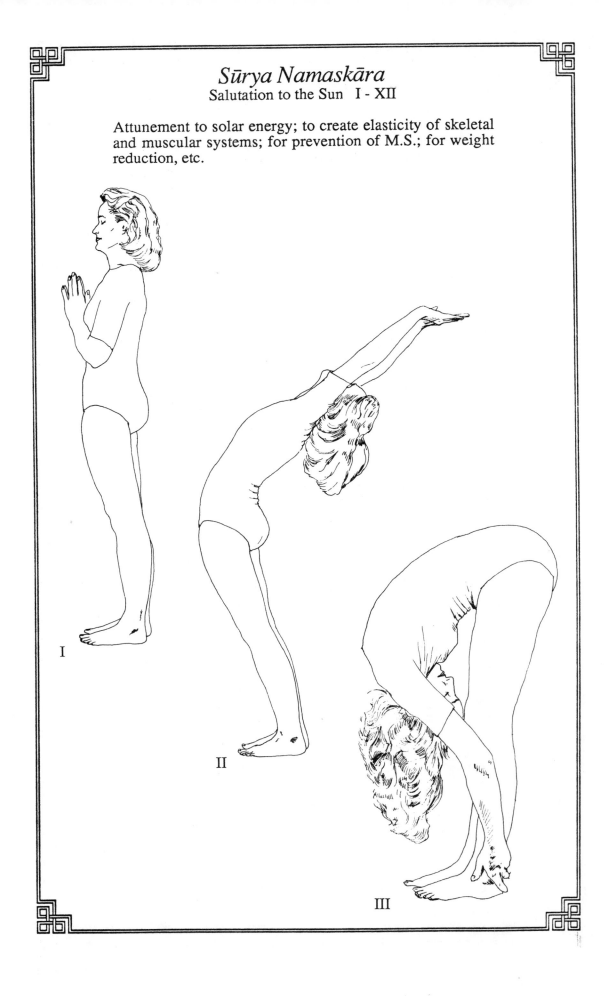

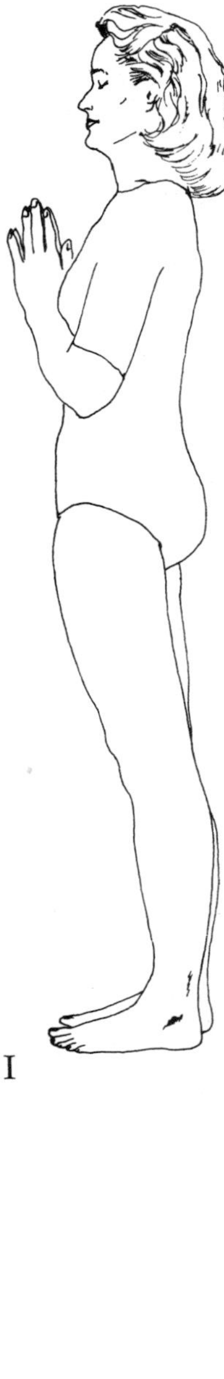

I

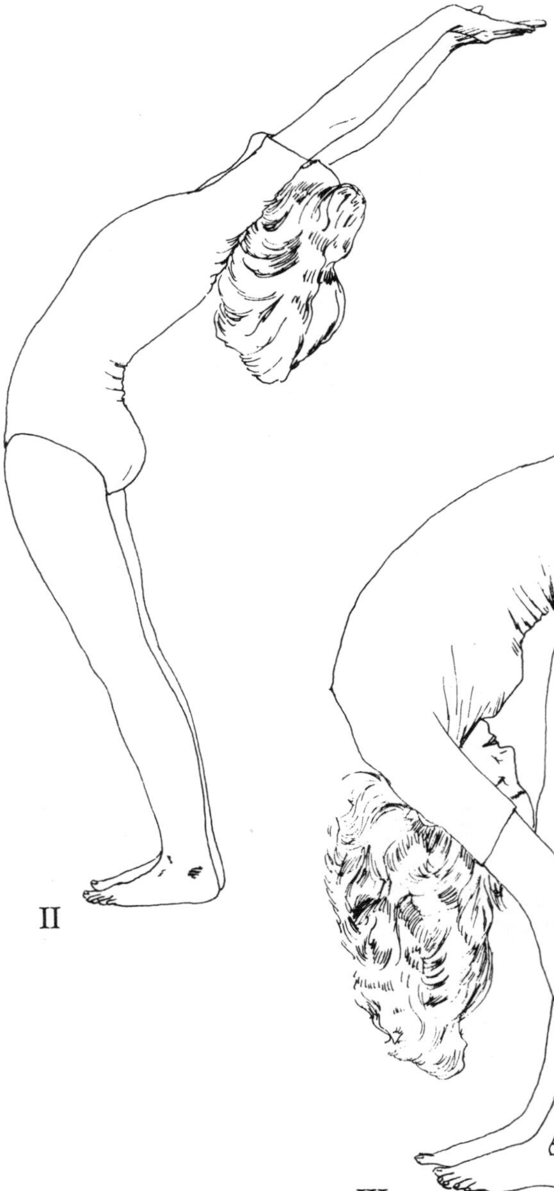

II

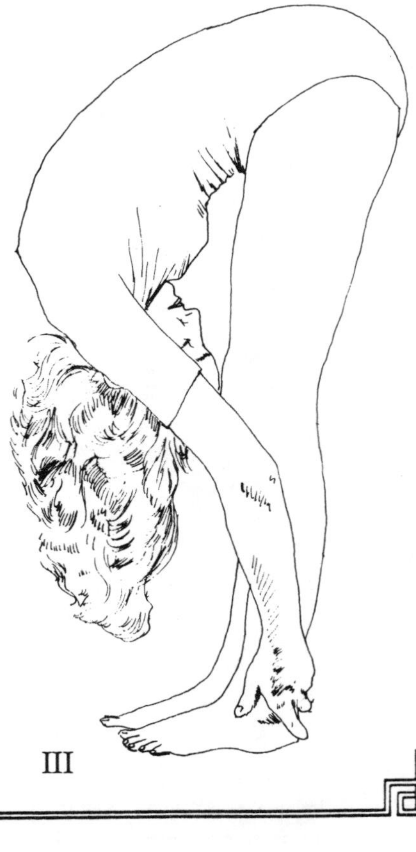

III

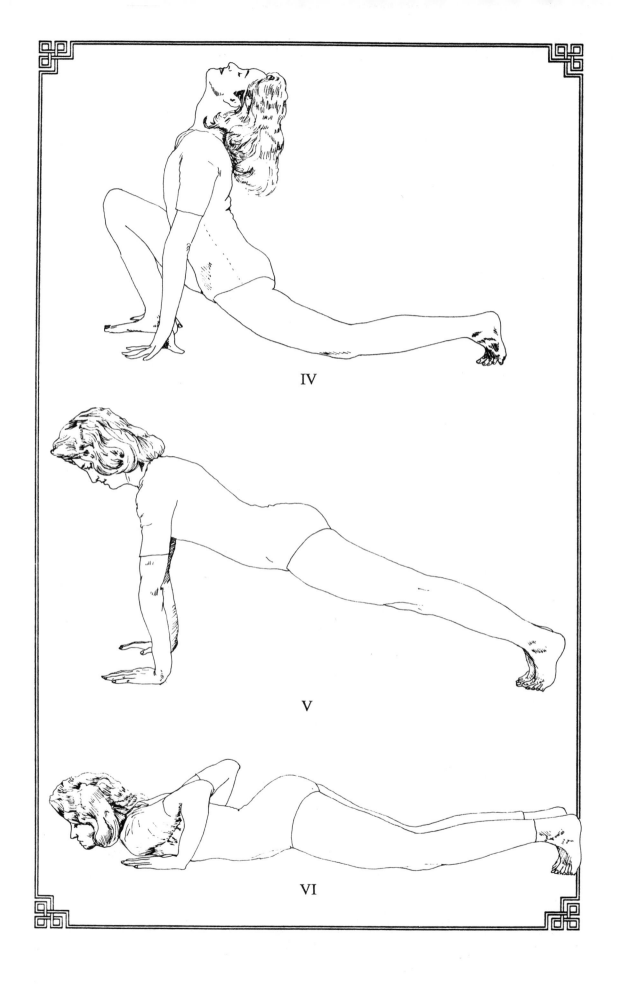

IV

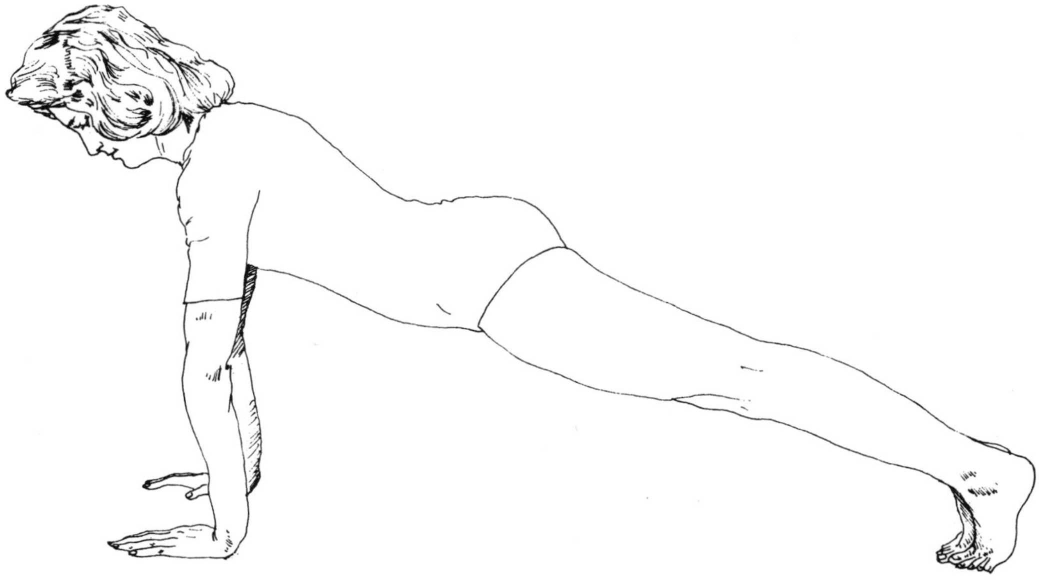

V

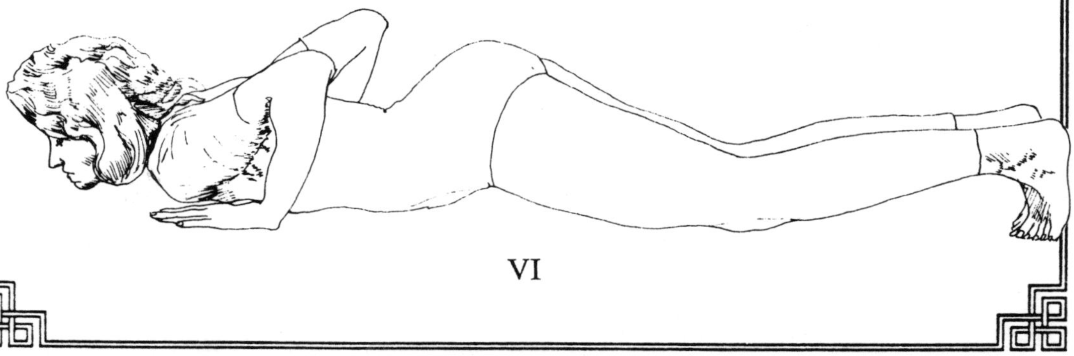

VI

Sūrya Namaskāra
Salutation to the Sun, cont'd.

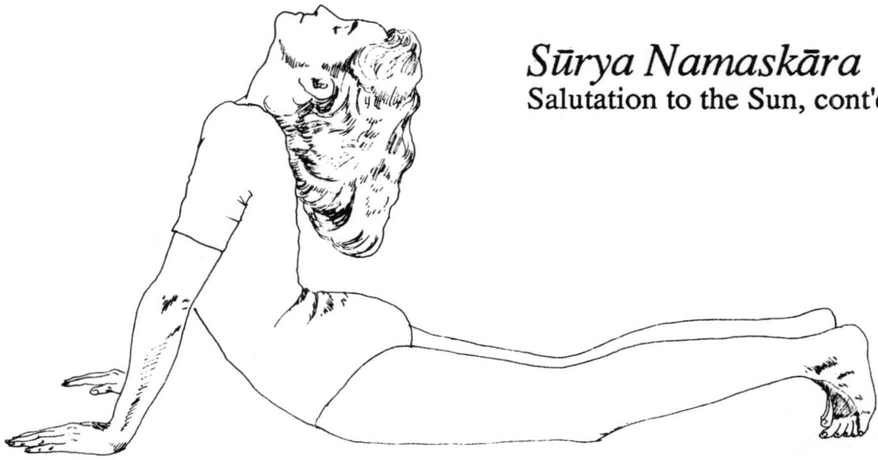

VII

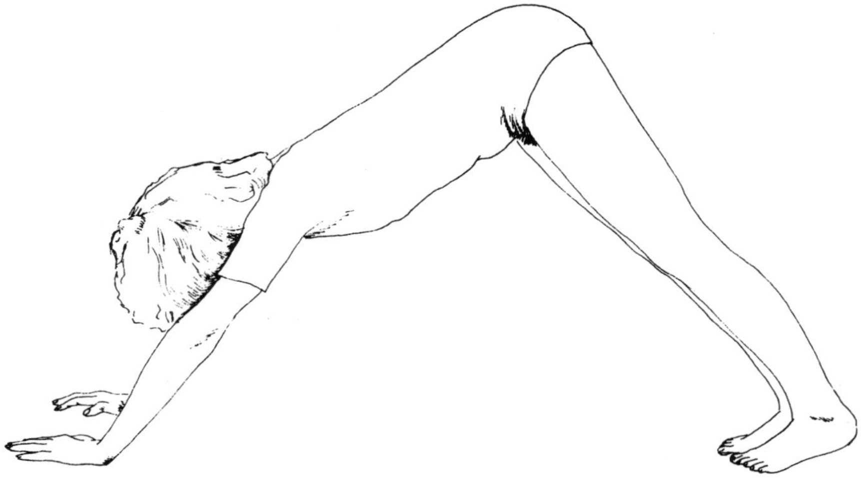

VIII

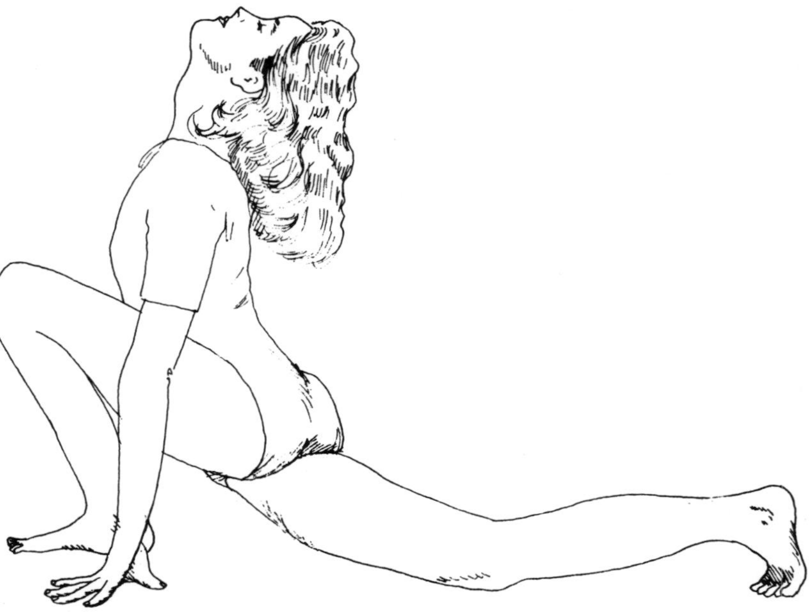

IX

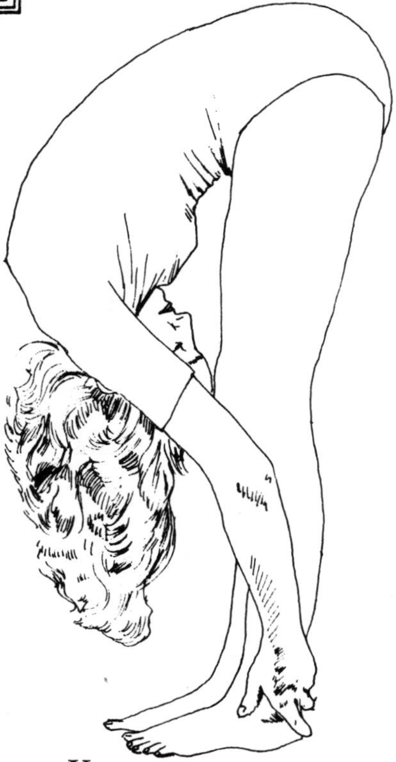

X

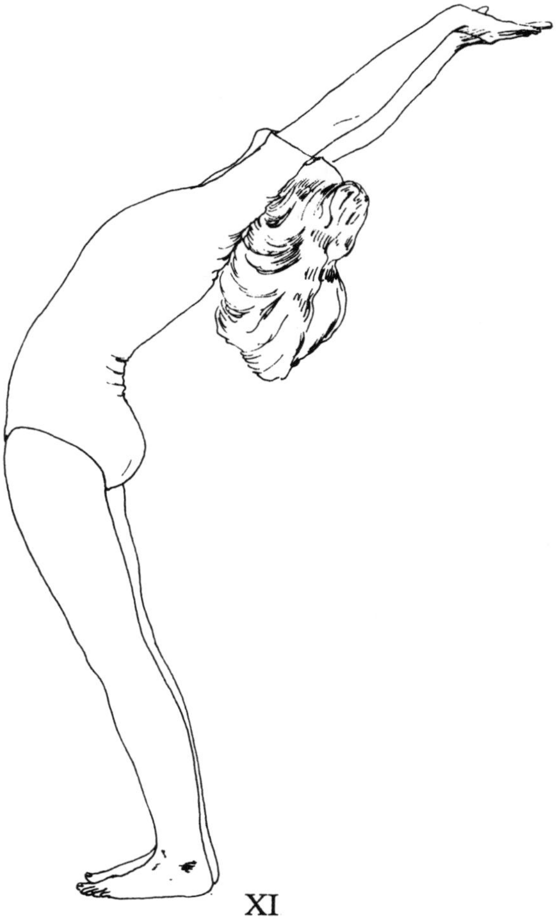

XI

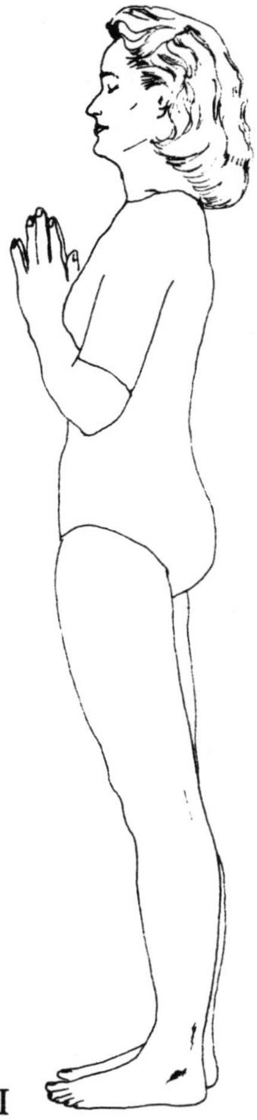

XII

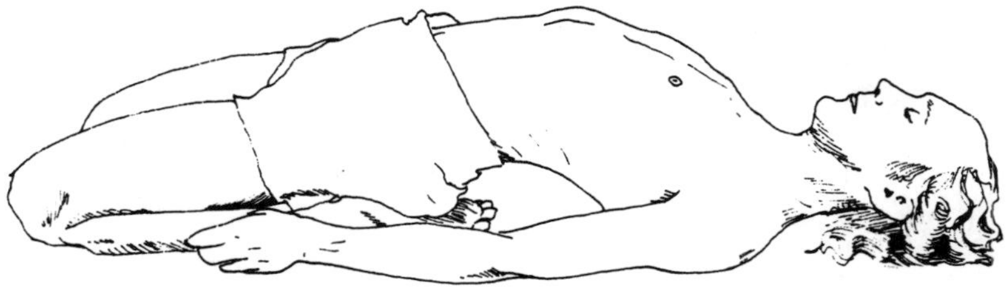

Supta Vajrāsana
Diamond pose, lying down

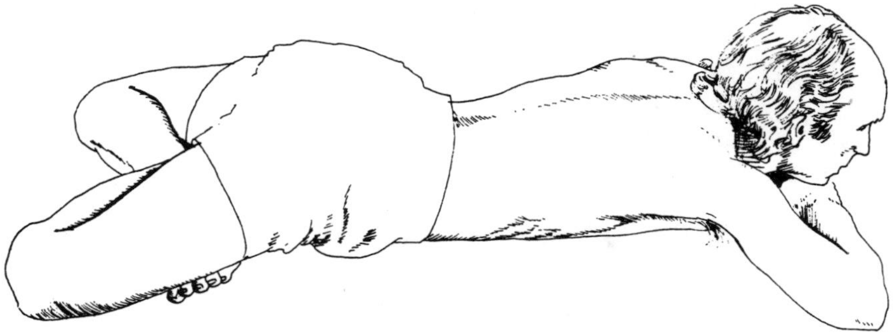

Matsyāsana, variation
Fish pose, variation

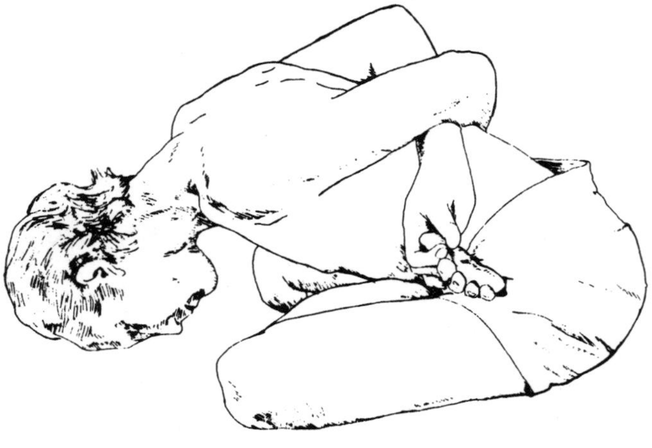

Baddha Padmāsana, variation
Bound Lotus pose, with forward bending

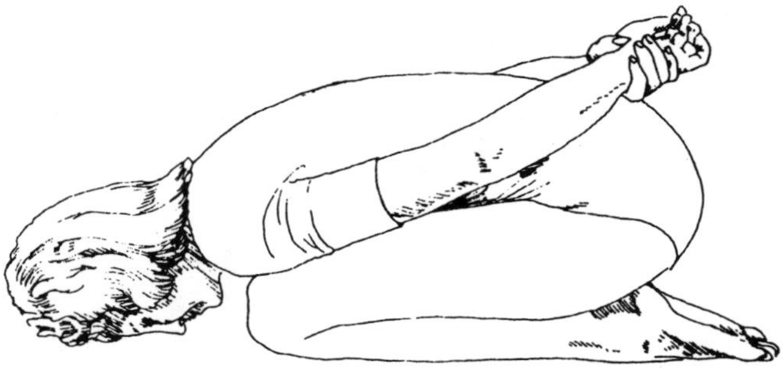

Yoga Mudrāsana I
Yogic Seal I

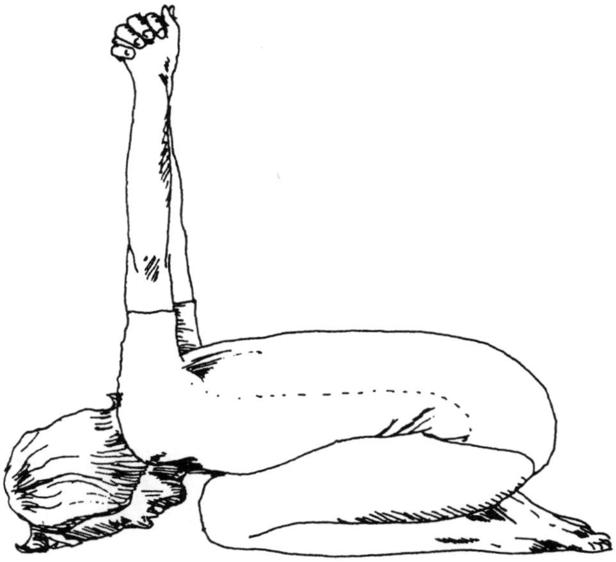

Yoga Mudrāsana II
Yogic Seal II

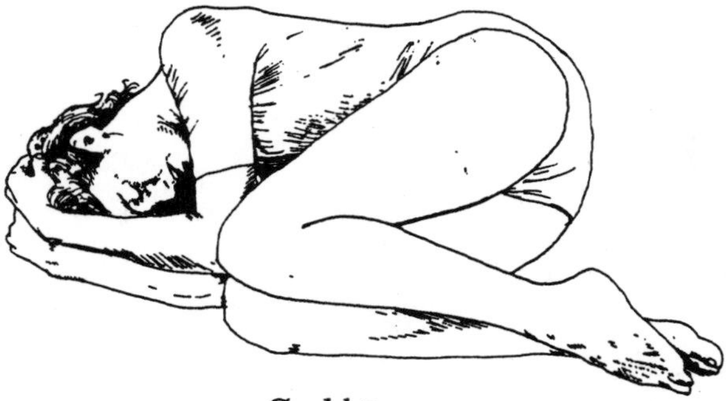

Garbhāsana
Fetus pose

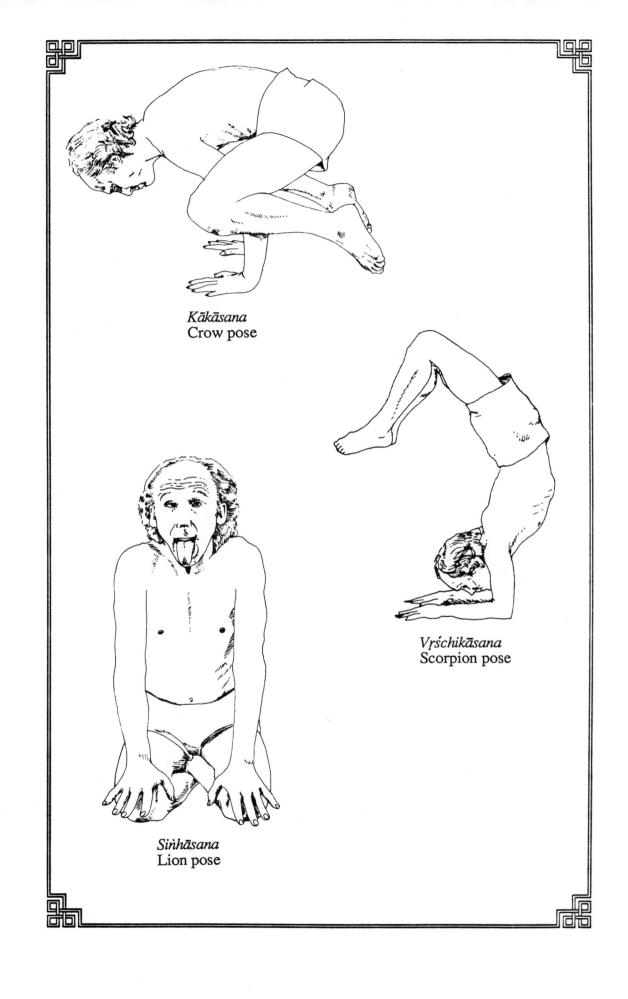

Kākāsana
Crow pose

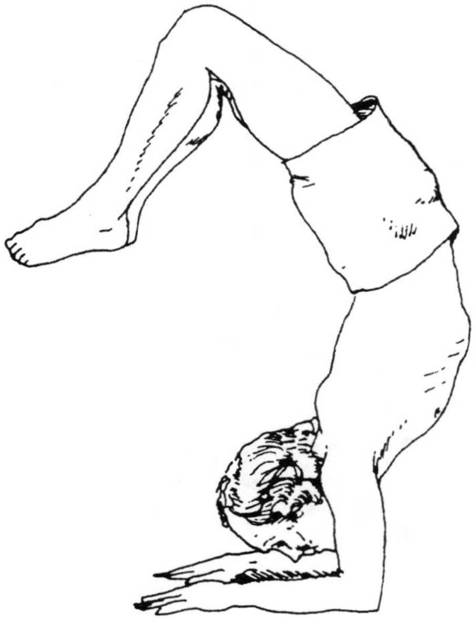

Vṛśchikāsana
Scorpion pose

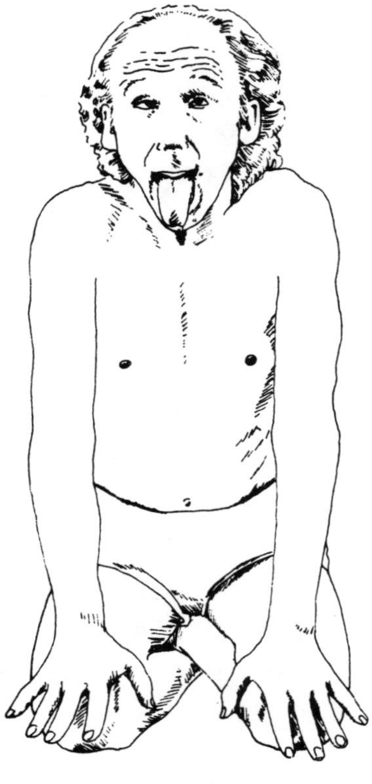

Siṅhāsana
Lion pose

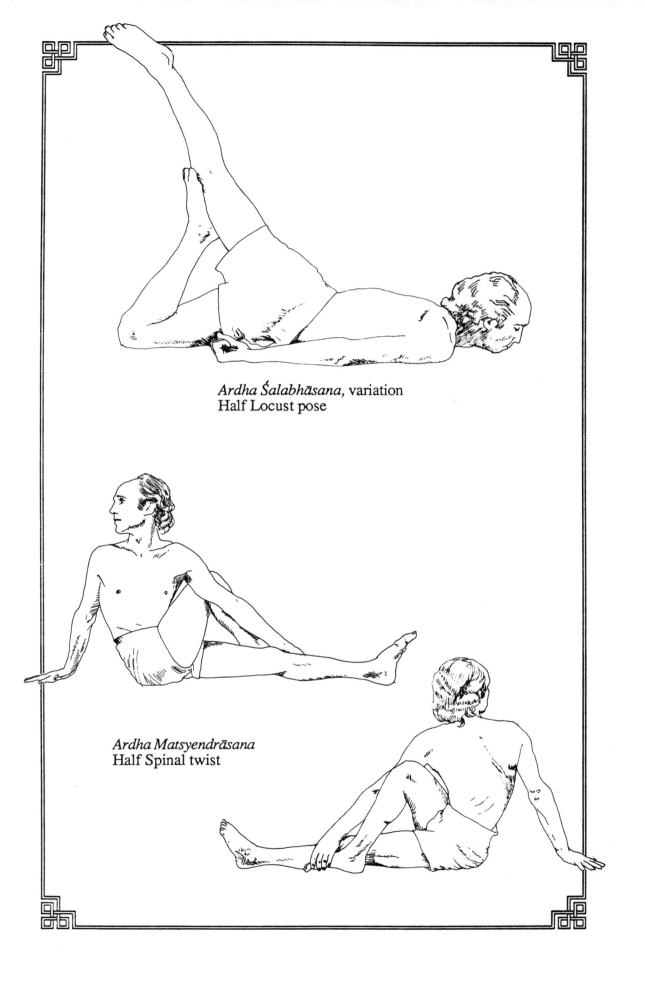

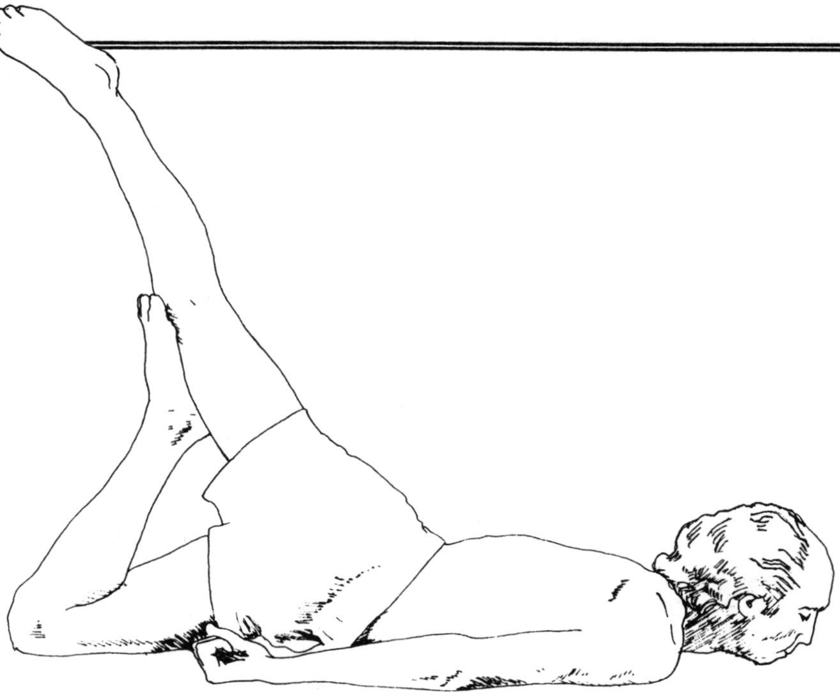

Ardha Śalabhāsana, variation
Half Locust pose

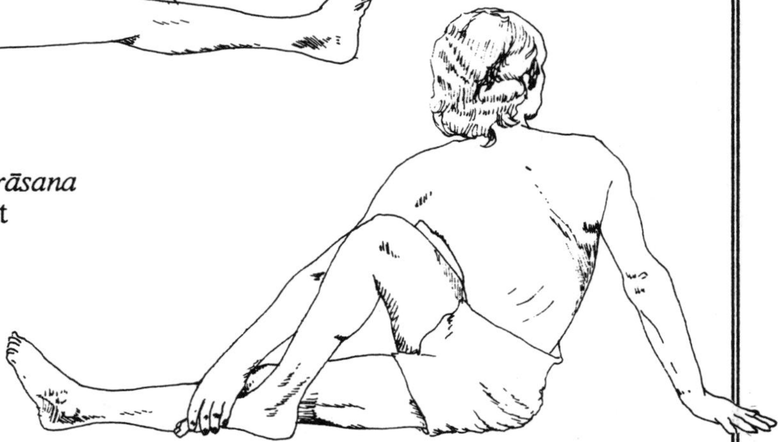

Ardha Matsyendrāsana
Half Spinal twist

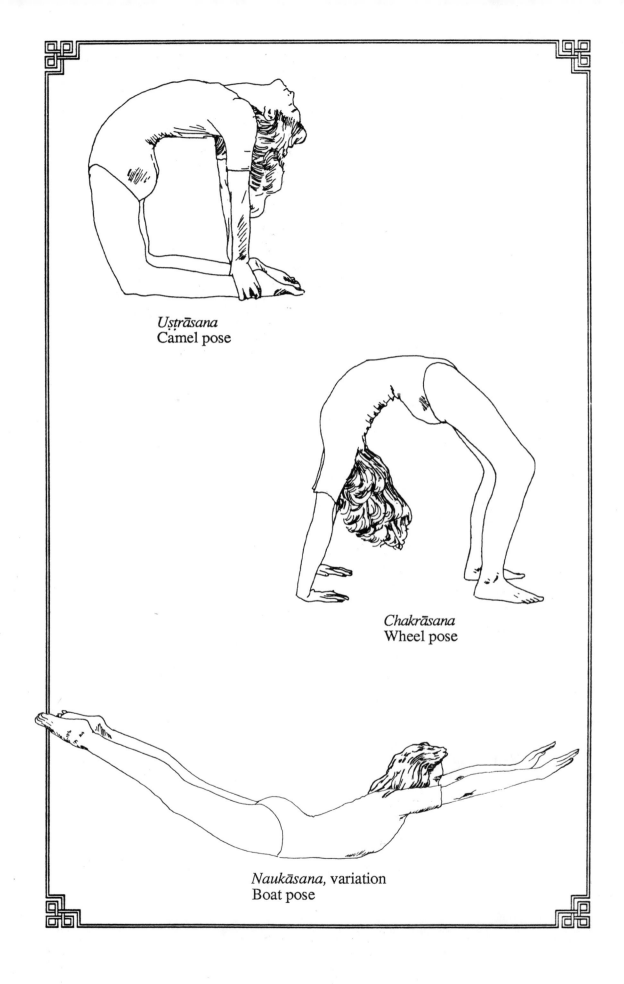

Uṣṭrāsana
Camel pose

Chakrāsana
Wheel pose

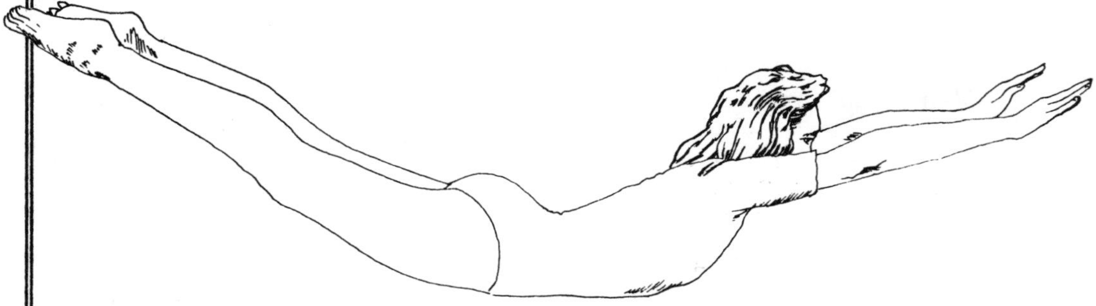

Naukāsana, variation
Boat pose

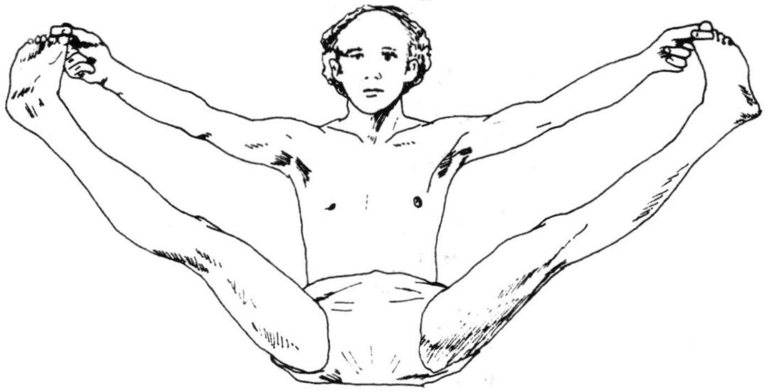

Vistṛta Pādāṅguṣṭhāsana
Expanded Hand-to-toes pose

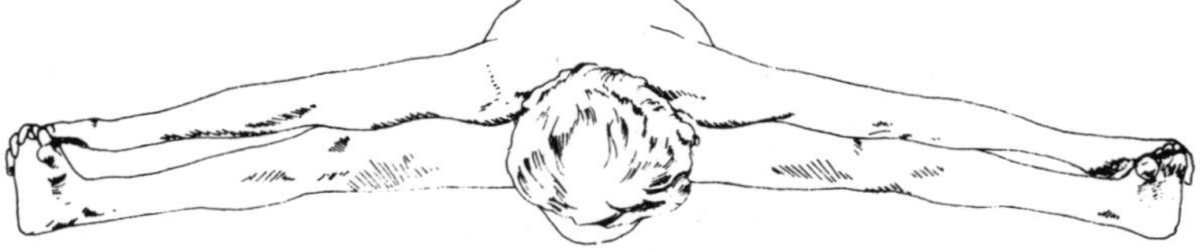

Upaviṣṭa Koṇāsana
Leg-and-arm stretch

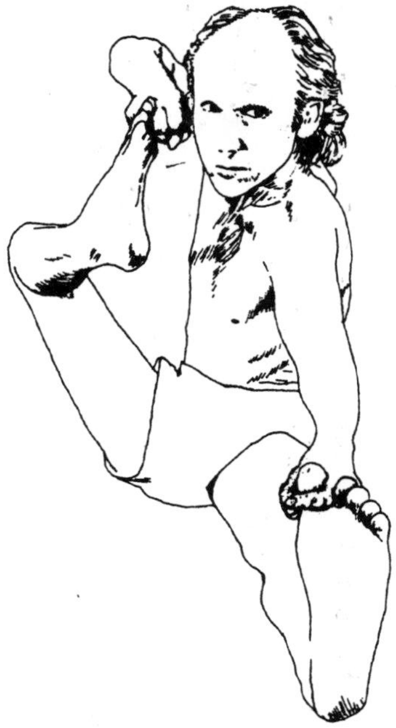

Ākarṇa Dhanurāsana
Shooting-bow pose

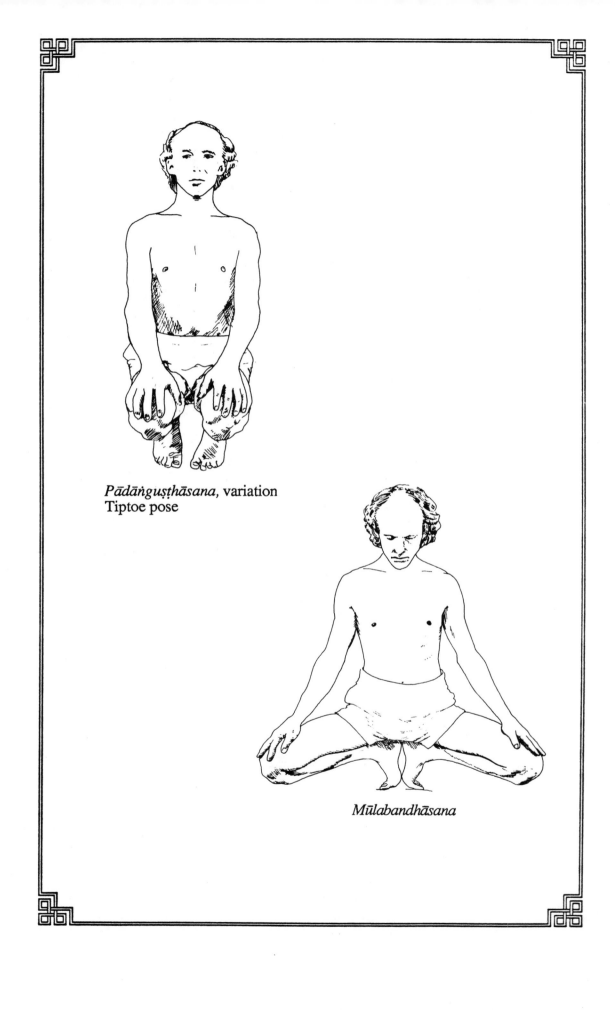

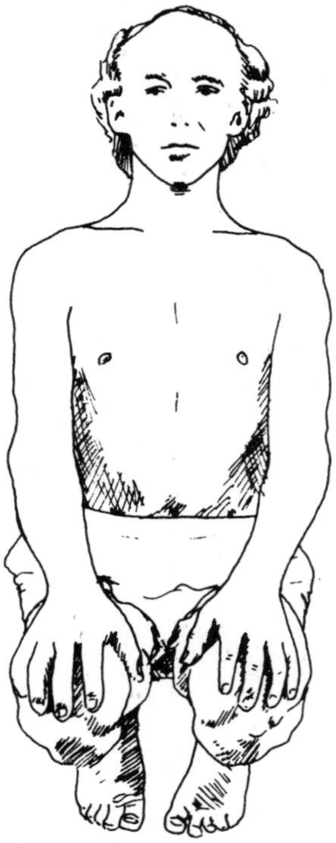

Pādāṅguṣṭhāsana, variation
Tiptoe pose

Mūlabandhāsana

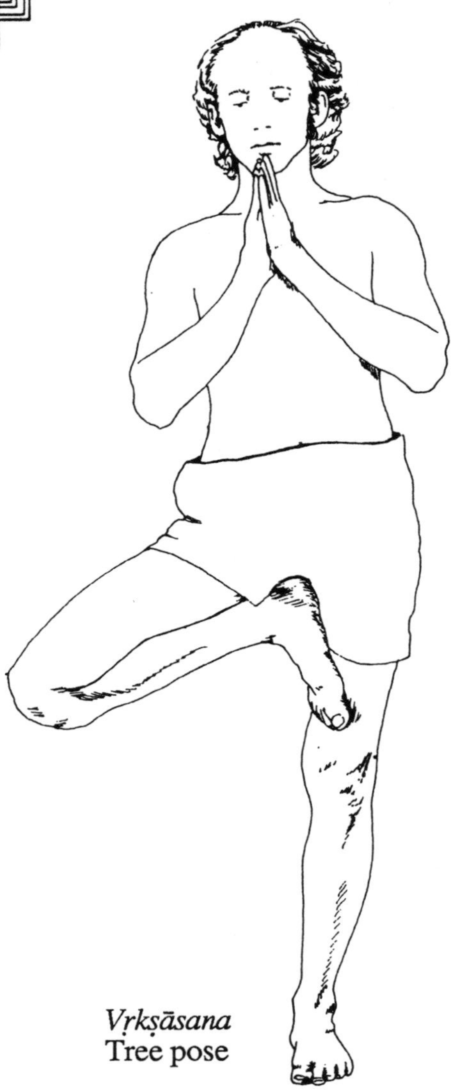

Vṛkṣāsana
Tree pose

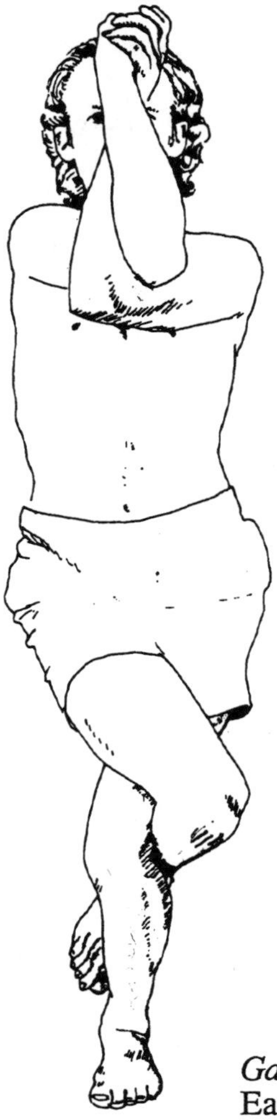

Garuḍāsana
Eagle pose

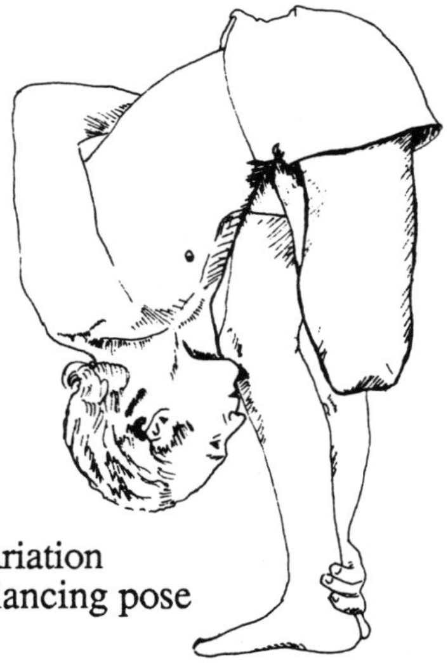

Jānuśīrṣāsana, variation
Head-to-knee Balancing pose

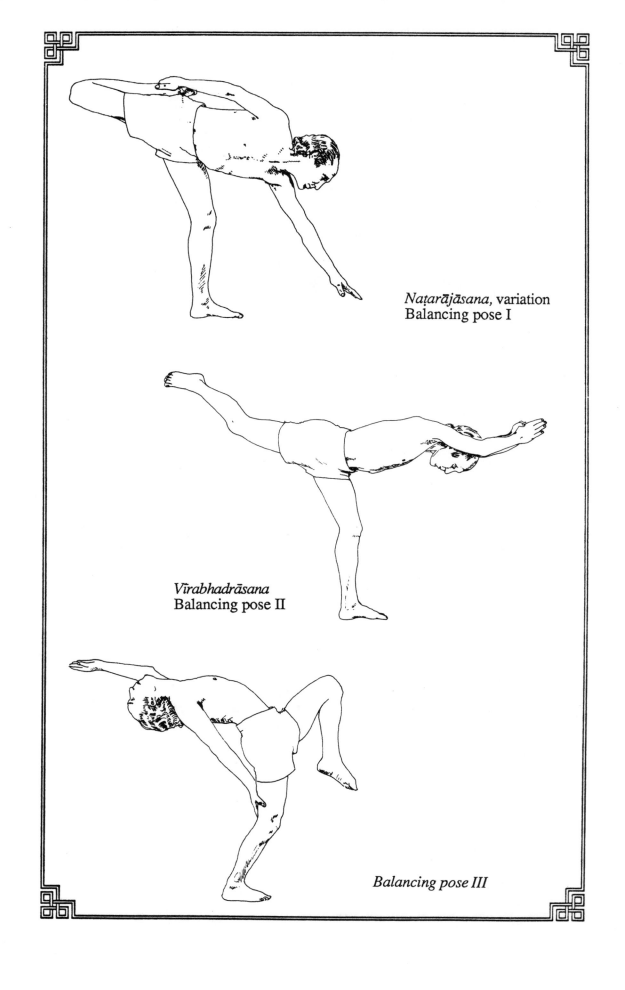

Naṭarājāsana, variation
Balancing pose I

Vīrabhadrāsana
Balancing pose II

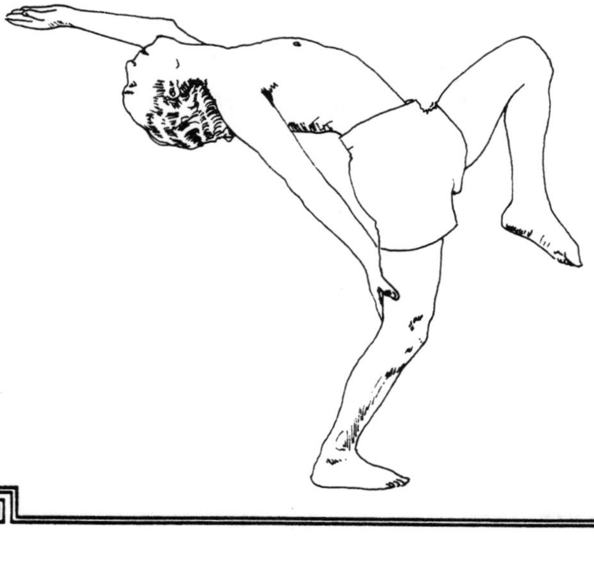

Balancing pose III

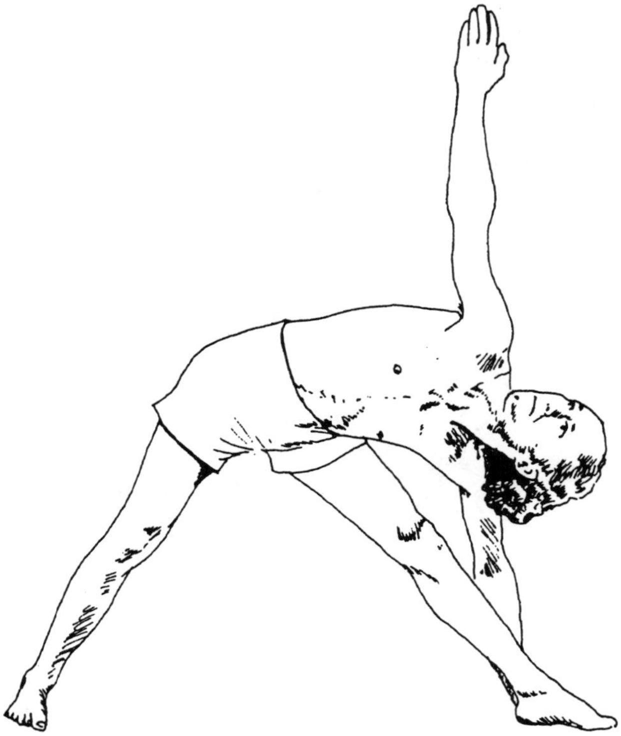

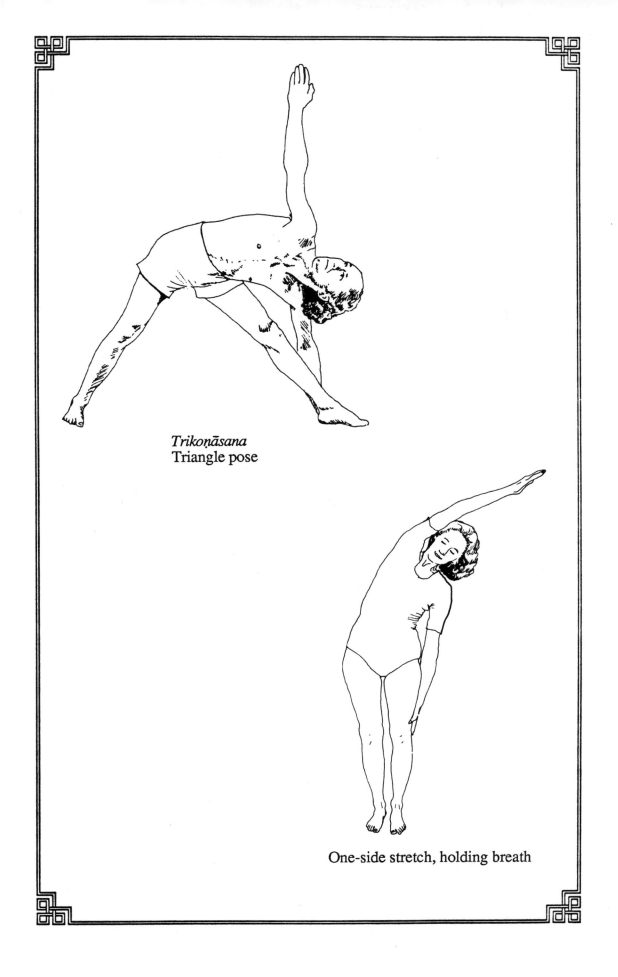

Trikoṇāsana
Triangle pose

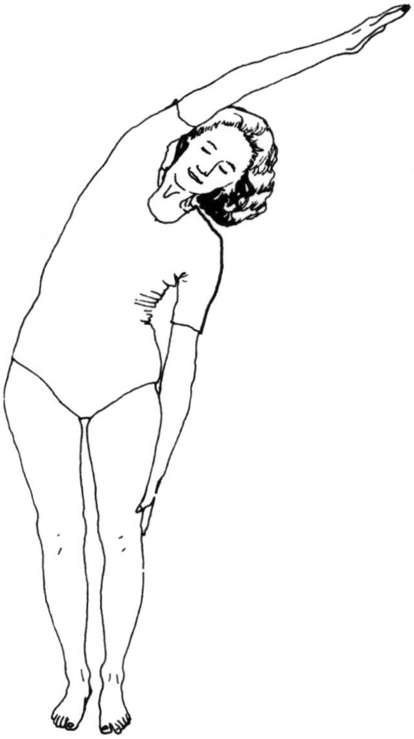

One-side stretch, holding breath

Śīrṣāsana

Headstand I - VIII

For balancing the force of gravity; for circulation of blood and electricity to the whole brain; for orientation in time and space.

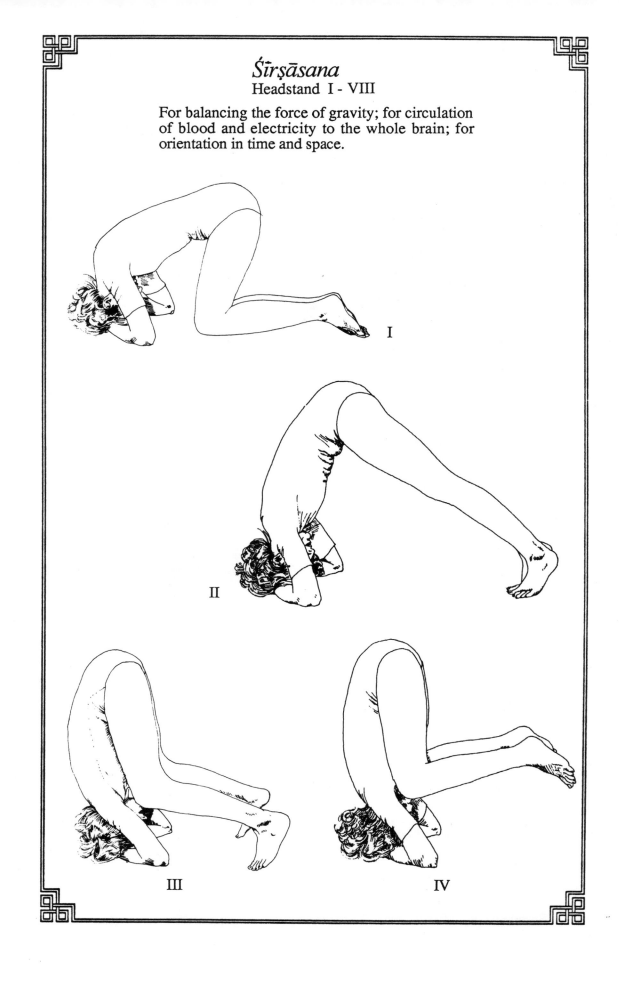

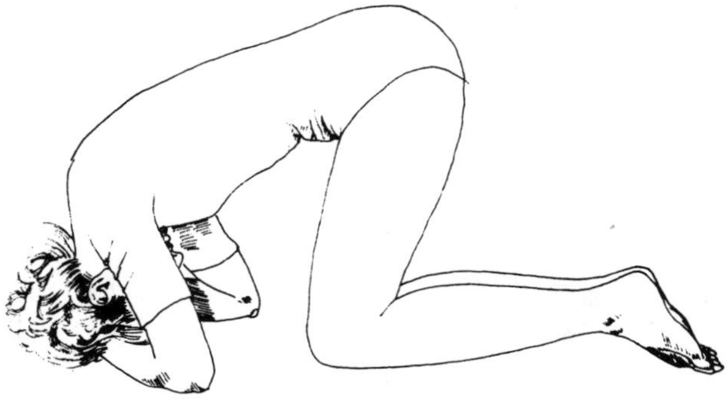

I

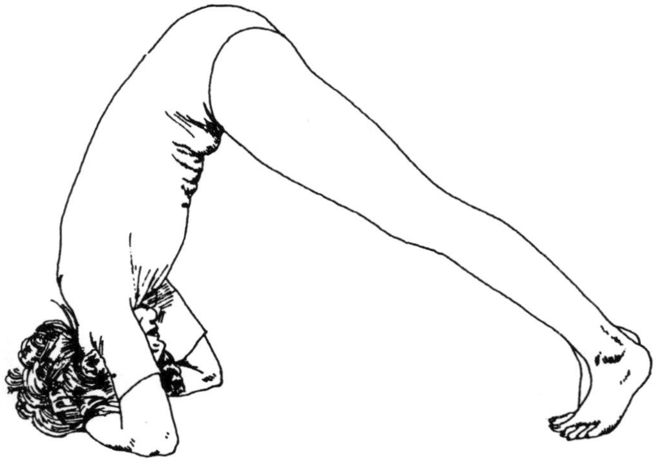

II

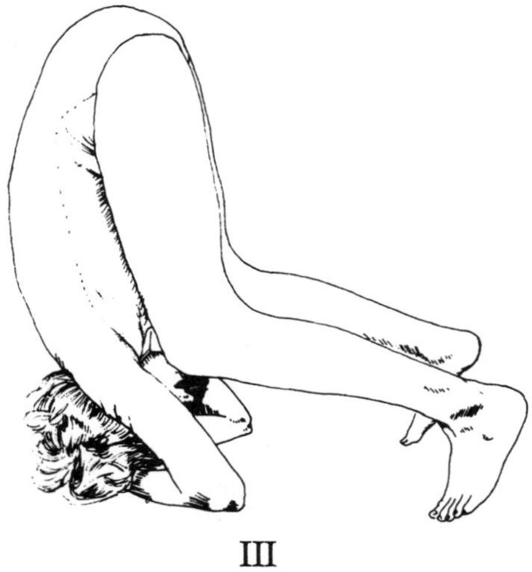

III

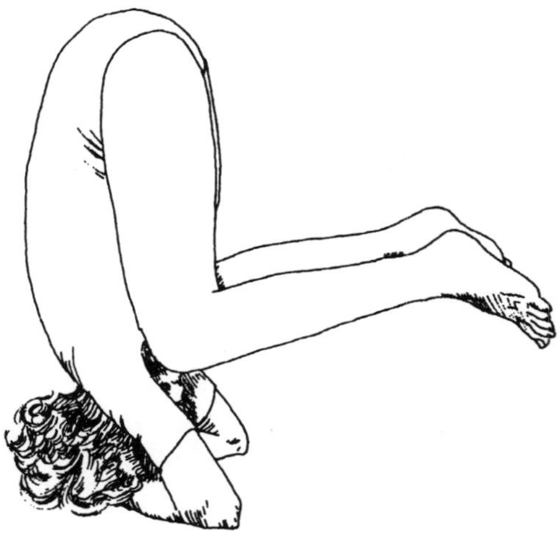

IV

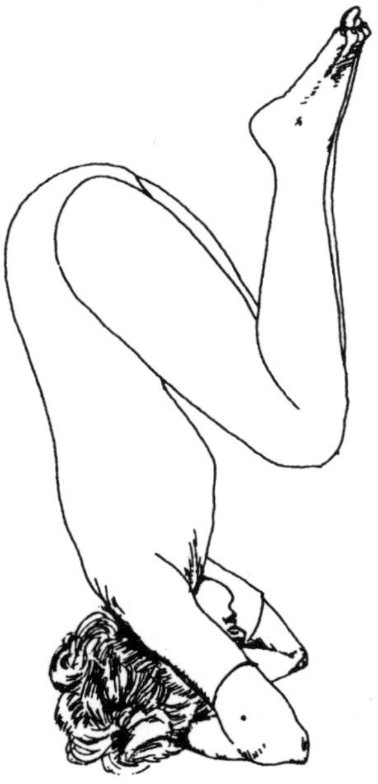

V

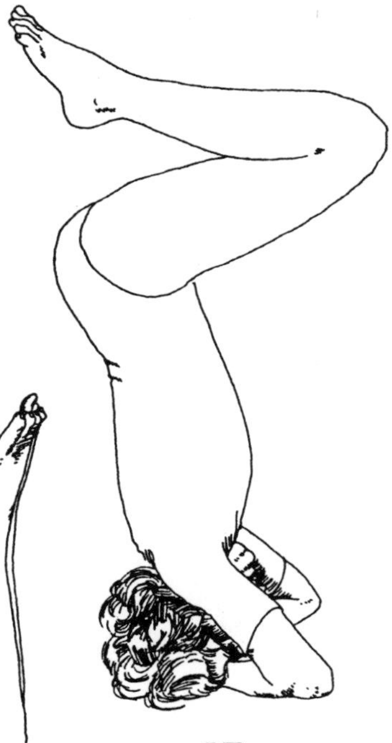

VI

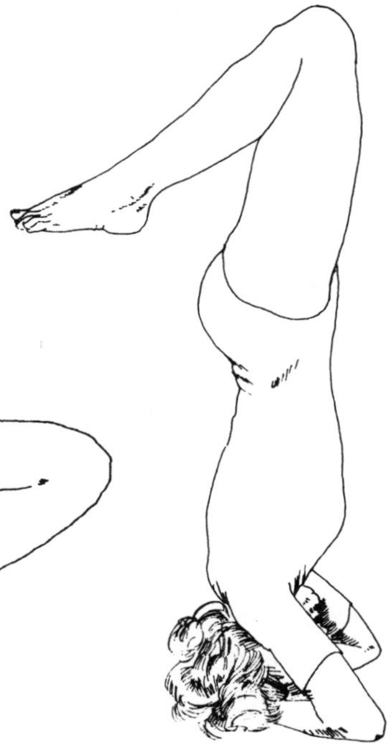

VII

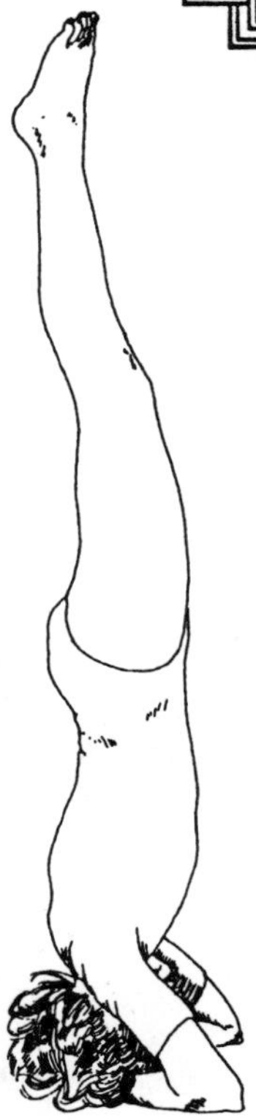

VIII

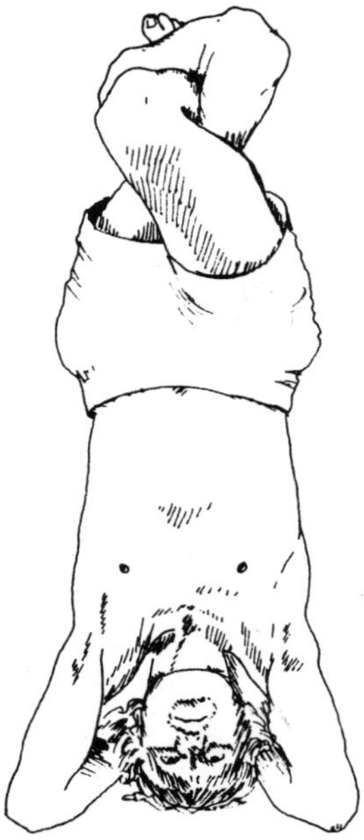

Śīrṣāsana, variation
Headstand Twist

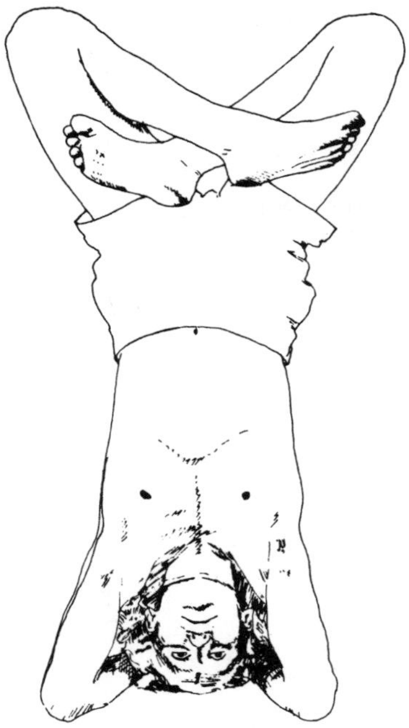

Ūrdhva Padmāsana in *Śīrṣāsana*
Upward Lotus pose in Headstand

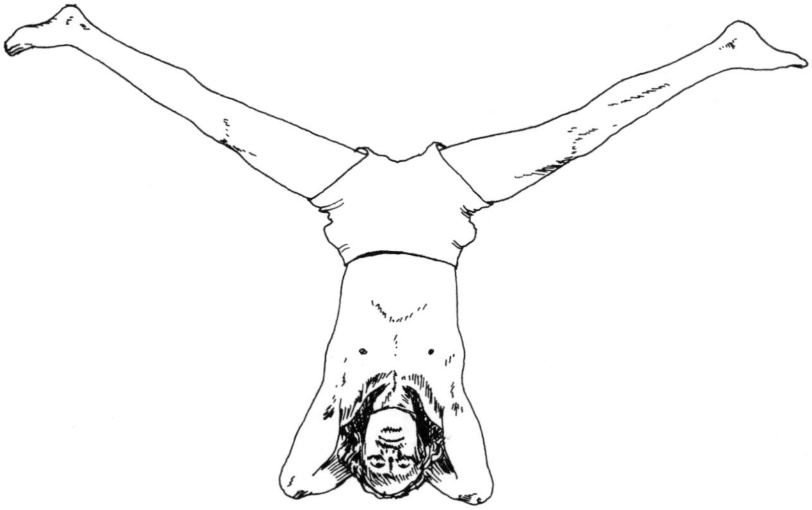

Vistṛta Pāda Śīrṣāsana
Headstand with legs spread

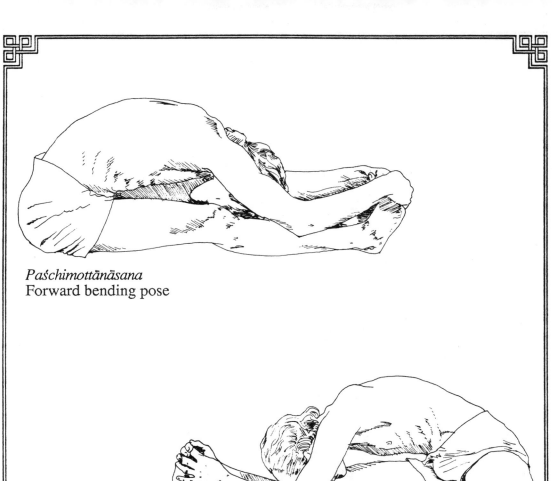

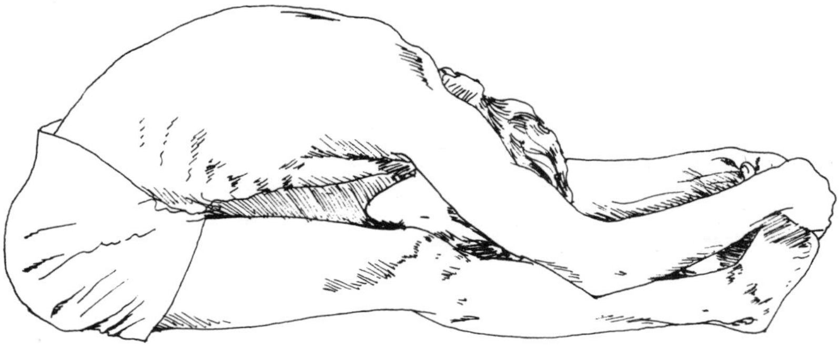

Paśchimottānāsana
Forward bending pose

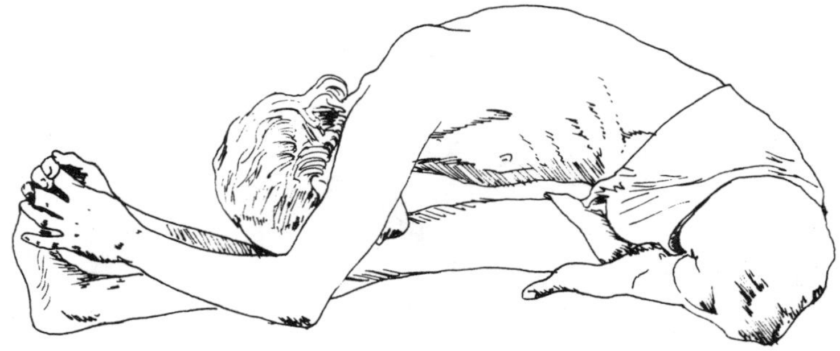

Jānuśīrṣāsana
Head-to-knee pose

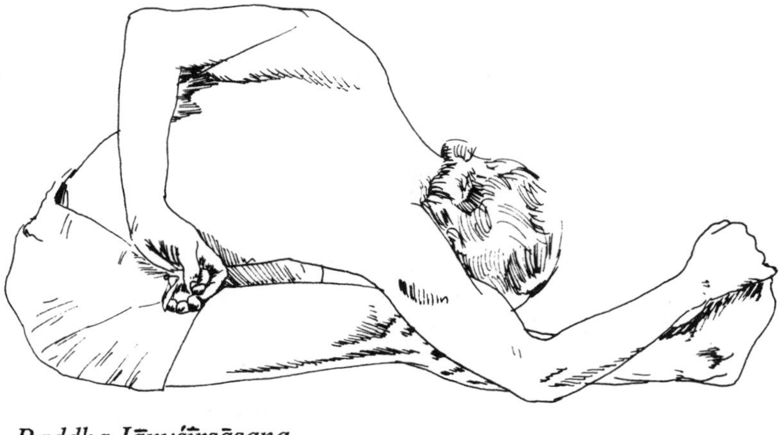

Baddha Jānuśīrṣāsana
Bound Head-to-knee pose

Crocodile Pose Series
(Spinal Twist) I - V

For the back and whole body; to prevent M.S.

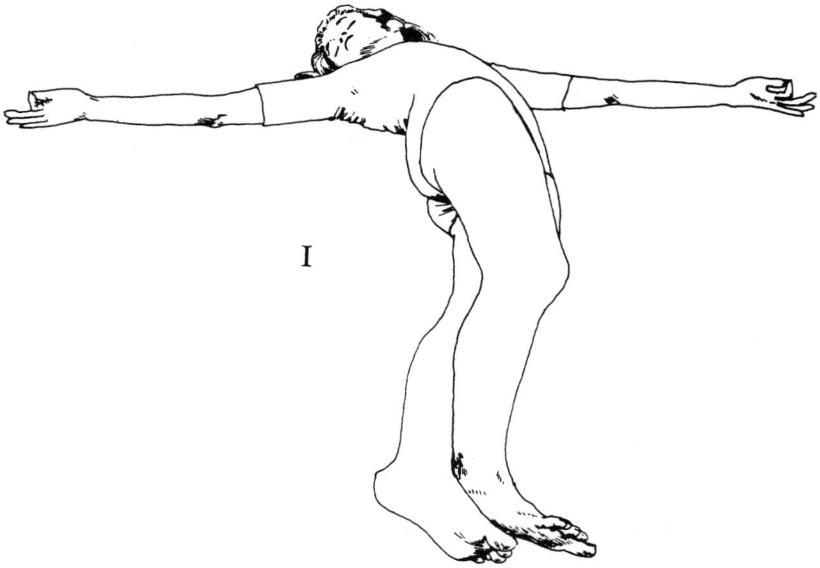

I

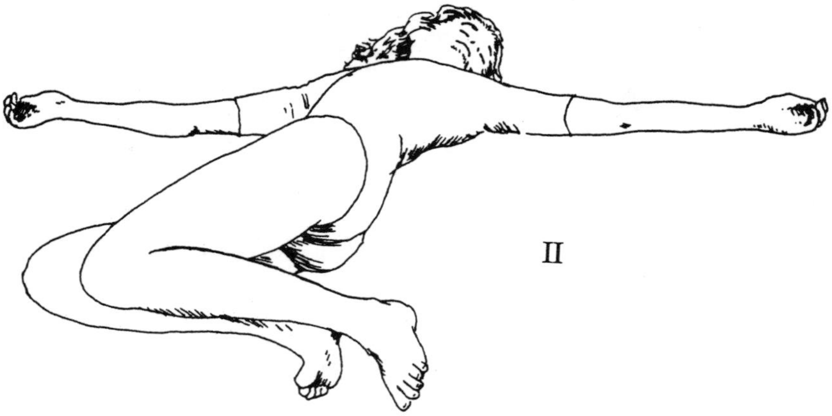

II

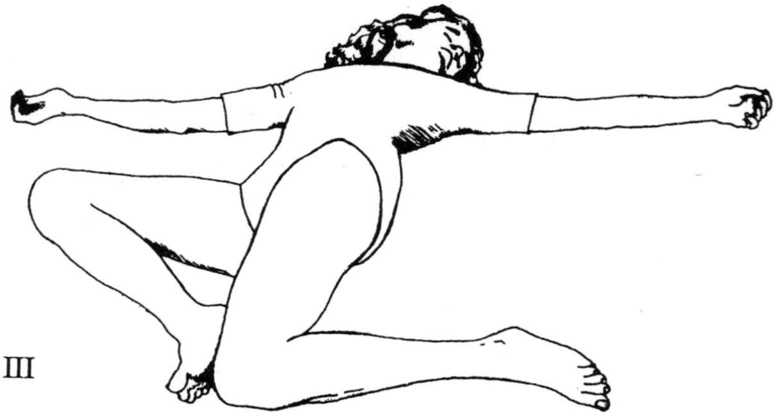

III

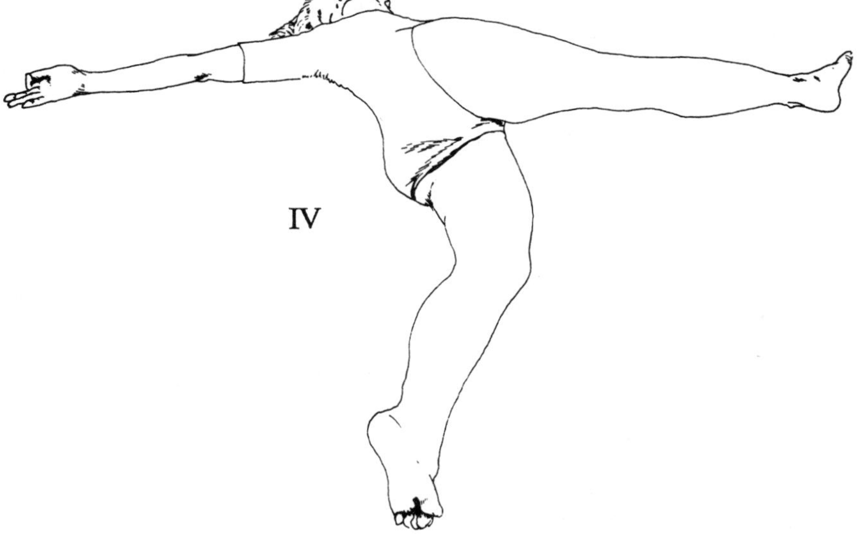

IV

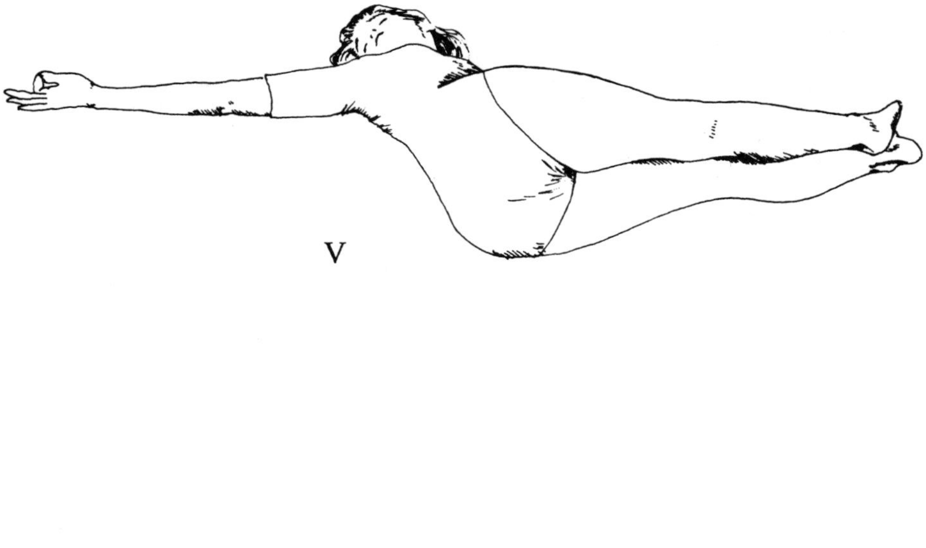

V

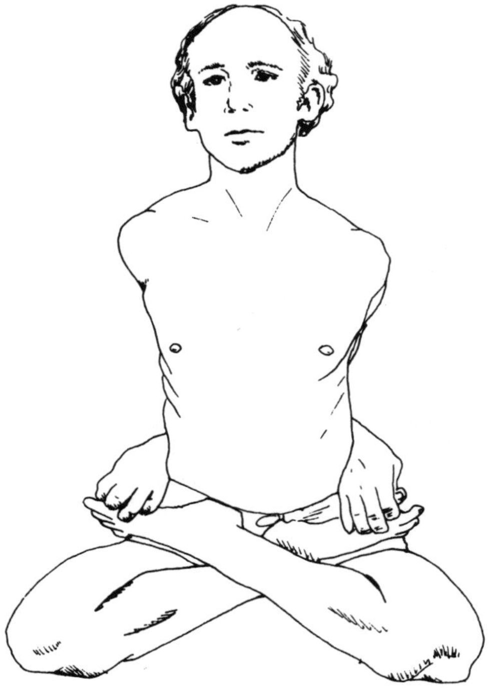

Baddha Padmāsana
Bound Lotus Pose

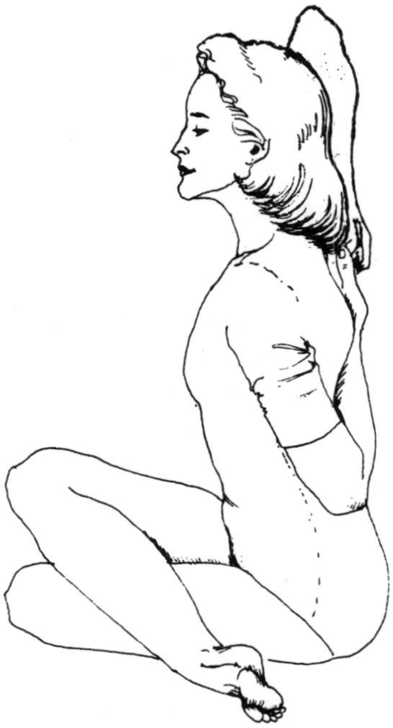

Gomukhāsana
Cow-head pose

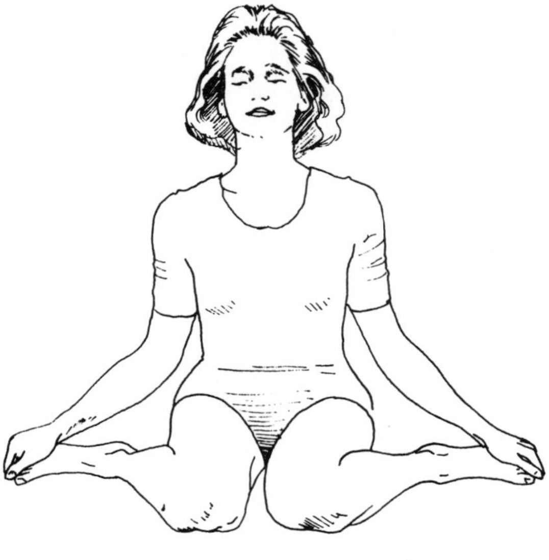

Gomukhāsana, variation
Leg stretch

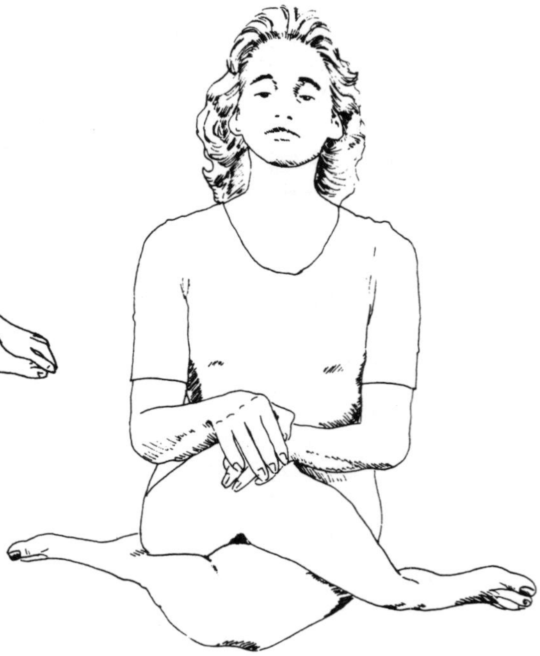

Vīrāsana
Heroic pose

GLOSSARY

abhyāntara vṛitti—that variety of *prāṇāyāma* in which the inhaled breath is held at maximal or near maximal lung capacity for as long as possible.

Aham Brahmāsmi—one of the great Vedic utterances used by a meditator as an aid in reaching the supreme state. It means "I am *Brahman*."

ahamkāra—universal ego, of which the individual sense of "I-ness" is a manifestation.

ahiṃsā—noninjury by body, speech, and mind, and the general attitude of welfare for the entire world. It is one of the yamas.

ājñā cakra(m)—the sixth of the seven *cakras*. It is located in the midbrain and is represented by the thalamus, which is the center of individual consciousness.

ākāśa—primordial nature, pervasive and the substratum of the entire material universe. Its most subtle manifestation is in the prenuclear state of matter, and it manifests as ether in the physical world.

anāhat(a)—the fourth of seven body *cakras* located in the region of the heart. This is a main seat of consciousness.

anāhat(a) nād(a)—manifestation in sound of the highest psychic energy (*prāṇa*) which may be heard in one form within the human body where it manifests at first close to the right ear.

ānandamaya—that sheath covering the Self which is composed of joy.

anātma vād(a)—the state of so-called "not self" in Buddhism. It is paralleled in Yoga by the experience of *asamprajñāta samādhi*.

anesthesia, yogic—the method of inducing complete relaxation of all or part of the body by means of *pratyāhāra* (withdrawal) and *dhyāna* (strong suggestion).

āpa—the liquid state of matter according to the *Sāṃkhya*-Yoga system.

apara vairāgyam—the first stage of renunciation in which one gains relative purity, detachment, and calm.

aparigraha—attitude of noncovetousness. It is one of the *yamas*.

ardha-matsyendrāsana—"the twist" posture of *Haṭha* Yoga.

arthana chandataḥ kriya—one of the eight supernatural powers gained by advanced Yogis. It involves being able to put into action whatever one wills.

asamprajñāta samādhi—the highest state of *samādhi* in which pure consciousness only is perceived and all distinctions between subject and object are lost. This is called the Absolute State and leads to complete liberation.

āsana—the third of the eight systems which comprise Yoga. In *Rāja* Yoga, the term means any comfortable position for meditation.

āśram—a fixed place of meeting where students advance themselves spiritually under the guidance of a teacher.

asteyam—vow of nonstealing. It is one of the five yamas.

ātman—term for the divine soul lying dormant in all living beings but able to be manifested to its fullest in man by the practice of meditation. It is variously called Self, Universal Principle, Supreme Consciousness.

aura and astral bodies—the various subtle manifestations of matter and energy which, in addition to the gross body, make up the abode of a human individual. These bodies are perceived only by those trained to see them.

aveśa—the power of entering into other bodies obtained by advanced Yogis.

ayamātmā Brahman—a Vedic suggestion repeated by the meditator as an aid in attaining the supreme goal of meditation. It means "This soul is *Brahman*".

bāhya vṛitti—the variety of *prāṇāyāma* in which the breath is forcefully exhaled and the lungs are held for a time at their lowest minimal air capacity.

bāhyābhyāntara visnayakṣepi—the most forceful of all *prāṇāyāmas* in which one makes multiple inhalations, one after another, without exhalation, until the lungs have reached absolute maximal capacity, and then multiple exhalations by the same process until the lungs have reached minimal capacity.

basti—one of six methods to purify and develop the body. It consists of cleansing of the bowels and sexual organs.

bhakti—complete devotion to and love for all beings because of the divine principle perceived in them through meditation.

bhāva pratyaya—the power of complete mastery of the physical world obtained through *asamprajñāta samādhi.*

bhāvasamādhi—the same as *samprajñāta samādhi.*

bherī nādam—the echo of chanted OM or any other sound which may be meditated upon.

bhrumadhya dṛiṣṭi—a form of *trāṭakam* in which the attention is fixed between the eyebrows.

bhūjangāsana—the *Haṭha* Yogic "cobra pose".

Brahman—the eternal, omnipresent, omniscient principle the realization of which is the goal of meditation. It is sometimes called Ultimate Reality because, although all is dependent upon it for existence, it is without relation, independent. It may also be defined as *Sat-cit-ānandam,* or Eternal Existence, Eternal and Complete Knowledge, and Highest Bliss.

Brahman bhāvanam—identification of one's self with Supreme Consciousness.

Brāhmī-sthiti—the perfect state where one becomes identified with *Brahman.*

buddhi—that principle of universal intuition to which the meditator becomes joined in the super-reflective state of *samādhi.* It lies latent in the human mind, above both intellect and ego.

cakras—seven subtle centers for consciousness symbolized in the human body by the areas at the base of the spine (*mūlādhāra*), the lumbar region (*svādhiṣṭhāna*), the solar plexus (*maṇipūra*).

— the heart (*anāhata*), the throat (*viśudhā*), the thalamus (*ājñā*), and the cerebral cortex (*sahasrāram*). Meditation usually takes place on the higher centers (*anāhata, ājñā,* and *sahasrāram*).

cetaśo jñānam—the power of telepathy gained by advanced Yogis.

cin nādam—any steady buzzing or whistling sound which may be concentrated upon.

cincin nādam—the roaring sound of a waterfall as an object of meditation.

citta prasādanam—serenity of the mind produced as a result of the practice of certain moral principles.

cittam—a technical term which means "seat of consciousness" and as such includes the conscious, subconscious, and superconscious minds. Yoga gives knowledge and control of the first two facets of *cittam* so that the third, or superconscious mind, may manifest.

dhanurāsana—the "bow posture".

dhāraṇā—the sixth of the eight systems which comprise *Rāja* Yoga. It consists of fixation upon the object of meditation and, as such, is the beginning of the internal stages of Yoga.

dhauti karm—one of six methods of physical cleanliness prescribed by Yoga. It is a means of cleansing the stomach by swallowing and removing a lengthy strip of gauze held on one end by the fingers.

dhyāna—the seventh of the eight systems making up Yoga. It is the intermediate internal process where the power of attention becomes so steadily fixed upon the object of meditation that other thoughts do not enter the mind at that time. This is the state properly called meditation. *Dhyāna* also includes the process of sending autosuggestions, such as to relax one's arm.

divya dr̥ṣṭi—the so-called "third" or "divine eye", located between the eyebrows or in *ājñā cakram.* This is the seat of intuition.

dualism—the perception of reality as two principles instead of one caused by the limiting properties of intellect and perceptual mechanism. Dualism disappears in *samādhi* where both intellect and senses are transcended.

eight systems—eight sets of practices which together comprise the science of Yoga. *Yama* and *niyama,* the first two steps, comprise the ethical foundation of Yoga: *āsana, prāṇāyām,* and *pratyāhāra* comprise means of physical preparation for the final internal practices of *dhāraṇā, dhyāna,* and *samādhi.*

ghaṇṭa nādam—the ringing sound of a bell which, if steady, may be meditated upon.

gunas—the three cosmic principles of which the entire material universe is composed in varying proportions. *Sato guṇa,* the first principle, manifests as life, light, freshness, resolution, good moral qualities, and, in the nuclear sphere, the proton. *Rajo guṇa,* the second principle, is characterized by activity and the electron. The characteristics of *Tamo guṇa* are sleep, dullness, decay, and the neutron.

guru—a teacher of the science of Ultimate Reality who, because of his extended practice and previous attainment of the highest states of meditation, is fit to guide others in their practice toward the same end.

halāsana—the plough pose.

Haṭha Yoga—a system of Yoga, developed later than *Rāja* Yoga, in which the various parts of the body were employed to effect control of the mind. An elaborate system of *āsanas* was developed and these have even more recently been employed for maintaining physical health as well as for spiritual progress.

heart—in beginning Yoga, that part of the body which, as the physiological symbol of *anāhata cakra,* sends life and electromagnetic pulsation to all parts of the body. It is a center for perceiving Universal Consciousness through pulsation to one advanced in meditation.

iḍa and *pingala*—Yogic terminology for the ascending and descending tracts of the autonomic nervous system. These pathways function in Yoga to open both subconscious and superconscious minds.

Īśvara—that conscious principle governing the entire physical universe.

jīvan mukta—the state of liberation while still retaining one's individual nature and physical body in order to do universal work for and in the world.

kaivalyam—same as *Nirvāṇam.*

kapala bhāti—one of six Yogic methods for physical cleanliness and health. It consists of a series of short, smooth inhalations and exhalations lasting up to the point of fatigue.

karma—that law of cause and effect which operates inexorably throughout the material universe. Also, a Yogic discipline in which one does all work and action unselfishly.

kośa—covering of the Self. It refers to any of the so-called "five sheaths" of body, *prāṇa,* mind, knowledge, and joy which limit manifestation of the Ultimate Reality.